NON-SURGICAL
TREATMENT OPTIONS FOR

# KNEE OSTEOARTHRITIS

NON-SURGICAL
TREATMENT OPTIONS FOR

# KNEE OSTEOARTHRITIS

An Informative Guide
for Patients

Ryan C. Koonce, MD

**OrthoSkool**
FOCUSED PATIENT EDUCATION

Copyright © 2019 Ryan C. Koonce, MD. All Rights Reserved.
Published by OrthoSkool Publishing

No part of this publication may be reproduced, stored in a retrieval system, or transmitted in any form or by any means, electronic, mechanical, photocopying, recording, scanning, or otherwise, except as permitted under the 1976 United States Copyright Act, without the prior written permission of the publisher.

ISBN: 978-1-7331358-1-8

### Limit of Liability / Disclaimer of Warranty

The information contained in this book is not intended to replace the advice of trained health professionals. This book represents the opinion of the author and this opinion may differ from that of other healthcare professionals. This book is not to be used to diagnose or treat any medical condition and it is not personal medical advice or recommendations. You are advised to seek the advice of licensed health professionals who are familiar with your individual health history and current health conditions to obtain information and education on your medical situation. You are solely responsible for the appropriateness and accuracy of your healthcare and you agree that you are using this book at your own risk. This book is sold "as is" and the author and publisher expressly disclaim all warranties. Reliance on the information provided in this book is for your own personal medical information, and the author and publisher expressly disclaim responsibilities for any and all errors, omissions, or inaccuracies associated with your use of this book. The author and publisher also expressly disclaim any and all personal, financial, or other risks incurred as a consequence, directly or indirectly, from the use and/or application of any of the contents of this book.

Published in the United States of America

Cover design by David Litwin / Pure Fusion Media

Cover image © [Sebastian Kaulitzki] / Adobe Stock

# Why You Should Read This Book

Nearly half of all adults will develop pain from knee osteoarthritis. Most of us don't want or need knee surgery, and there are lots of non-surgical treatment options available.

But which options are best for you? Remedies for knee pain are advertised in magazines, radio ads, billboards, and television. Which are legitimate and backed by science? Which are myths? There is a lot of snake oil being sold by so-called "experts". Knowing who to trust and how to navigate the medical system are significant challenges for today's consumers. We are faced not with a lack of information, but rather, information and marketing overload.

The goal of this book is to provide quality, science-based, and easy-to-understand information on available treatments for knee osteoarthritis. If this is what you are seeking, you've found the right resource.

Also by Ryan C. Koonce, MD:

*YOUR KNEE REPLACEMENT*
*A Patient's Guide To:*
*Understanding Hip Arthritis*
*Preparing for Surgery*
*Maximizing Your Outcome*

*YOUR HIP REPLACEMENT*
*A Patient Guide To:*
*Understanding Hip Arthritis*
*Preparing for Surgery*
*Maximizing Your Outcome*

*NON-SURGICAL TREATMENT OPTIONS*
*FOR KNEE OSTEOARTHRITIS*

*NON-SURGICAL TREATMENT OPTIONS*
*FOR HIP OSTEOARTHRITIS*

———————————

For online joint replacement education, check out:
www.OrthoSkool.com

**OrthoSkool**
FOCUSED PATIENT EDUCATION

# Contents

| | | |
|---|---|---|
| Chapter 1 | **Introduction** | 1 |
| Chapter 2 | **Basics of Knee Arthritis** | 7 |
| Chapter 3 | **Lifestyle Changes** | 19 |
| Chapter 4 | **Physical Therapy and Complementary Therapies** | 25 |
| Chapter 5 | **Injections** | 32 |
| Chapter 6 | **Medications and Supplements.** | 40 |
| Chapter 7 | **Topical Creams, Lotions, and Ointments** | 48 |
| Chapter 8 | **Braces and Assistive Devices** | 50 |
| Chapter 9 | **Where to Go from Here** | 54 |

Appendix

**Strength Exercises for Knee Arthritis** ........ 57

**Stretching Exercises for Knee Arthritis** ........ 63

**Other Resources** ........ 65

Glossary ........ 66

Image Credits ........ 73

Selected References ........ 74

*To Gavin, who constantly reminds me of the power of laughter and the privilege of being a father. You are my best buddy. Forever.*

# Acknowledgments

I sincerely appreciate the many surgeons who patiently trained me in the science and art of orthopedic surgery. To the surgeons at the University of Colorado, who reinforced the critical concept of putting patients first, and later welcomed me home as a colleague. To the surgeons at San Diego Sports Medicine and Arthroscopy Fellowship, who showed me the joy in caring for active patients. To the surgeons at the renowned Anderson Orthopaedic Clinic, who humbled me with their knowledge, inspired me with their intellect, and shared their exceptional surgical techniques. Thank you doesn't cover it.

Lastly, thank you to the patients, past and future, who put their trust in me as their surgeon. It is an honor and a privilege to be part of your joint replacement journey.

Chapter One

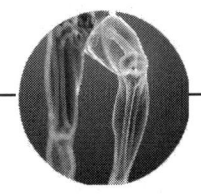

# Introduction

Don had always loved the outdoors and considered himself a "mountain man". His leisure time was a steady mix of hiking, camping, fishing, skiing, and rock climbing. Don worked as a field biologist, which, to his delight, supplemented his time in the outdoors. He considered the wilderness of Colorado his health club and his active lifestyle kept him feeling young and vibrant.

During one of his summer backpack trips, noticed pain in his left knee. It wasn't severe, and it didn't stop him from venturing outdoors, but he had to admit it was slowing him down. In the midst of summer, Don couldn't allow knee pain to get in the way of his hobbies or work. Eventually, he booked an appointment with me and his evaluation showed osteoarthritis in the left knee.

Don had no desire for surgery given his relatively mild symptoms and busy summer schedule. I agreed that jumping into surgery would be a bit hasty, so we discussed a few simple treatment options for him to try. We discussed that not every treatment works for every patient, and he selected a few that he was comfortable trying out.

This new diagnosis opened up the floodgates of advice from his neighbors and friends. His family sent him information on new injections and supplements that they heard cured knee arthritis. As a man of science, Don was skeptical about quick fixes. He returned to see me, and we discussed which options are backed by quality research and which are not.

Don's story and questions are common. Navigating the multitude of available treatment options for knee arthritis can be confusing. This book is written for patients who have knee arthritis, questions about their condition, and are seeking a reliable source of information that outlines the best non-surgical treatment options.

## Individualizing Treatment Plans

If you have knee pain or knee arthritis, there are dozens of advertised treatment options. The choice of treatment depends on many factors; some depend on the patient and some depend on the medical practitioner. A single patient could visit several types of medical practices and be offered many different treatments for the SAME knee condition. If medical practitioners disagree on the optimal treatment, how are patients to digest the vast amount of information available and participate in deciding for themselves?

Even after reading this book, there will not be ONE simple solution that suits every patient's needs. The BEST treatment depends on your genetics, biology, health history, activity levels, and your specific condition. The purpose of this book is to arm you with knowledge and background to assist with making an informed decision after discussing your specific needs with your medical practitioner.

## Science Versus Myths

In medical school, aspiring doctors are taught how to evaluate scientific papers not only for what they conclude, but HOW those conclusions are reached. Well-designed and well-executed scientific studies are the most meaningful. In order to be published in a medical journal, studies are typically reviewed by experts in a field. This is what is meant by *peer-reviewed* journal articles. Amongst peer-reviewed articles, there is a spectrum of quality. The quality of published studies varies from journal to journal.

The medical and scientific communities have established rating systems called "levels of evidence" that play some role in determining how meaningful a study's results are (Figure 1-1). The king of studies is the *randomized control trial*, whereby the researchers take a treatment, randomly assign that treatment to a group of patients, and gave an alternative or treatment to other patients, and analyze the results. On the other end of the spectrum, the lowest recognized level of evidence is *expert opinion*. Expert opinion is typically only accepted when higher levels of evidence are sparse or not available for a scientific question, and the person giving the opinion is a recognized name or leader in that field of science.

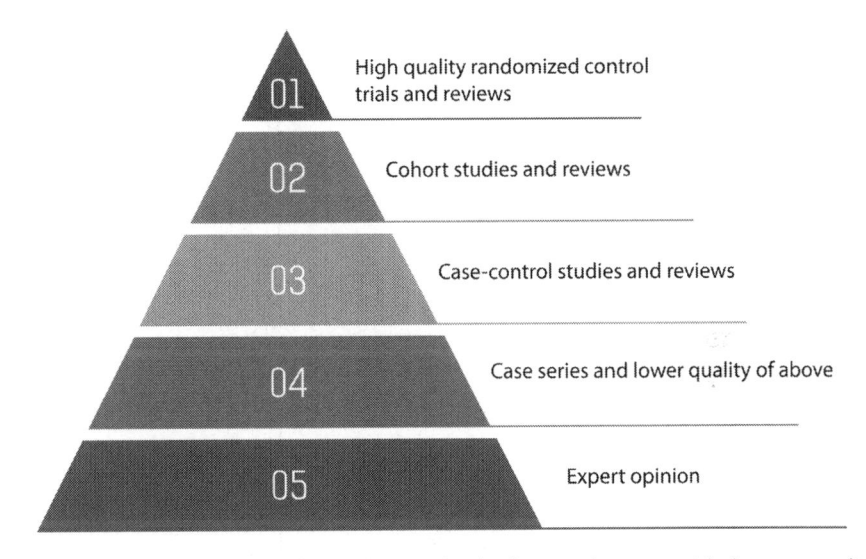

**Figure 1-1**: Levels of scientific evidence—the higher on the pyramid, the more valid the results of a scientific study. Note that anecdotal evidence and patient testimonies are not on the pyramid.

It has been my experience that if a treatment is safe and effective for treating a medical condition, the scientific community will study it properly. Despite this, treatments that lack verifiable scientific evidence to support their use but are still used by patients and some medical practitioners. Until a treatment is proven definitively to work, it's what I consider a *myth*. Just like other myths in society, these treatment myths lack a foundation in science.

Treatment myths are often formed based on *anecdotal evidence*. This is the evidence that a single practitioner or group might use to decide what treatments work for their patients in the absence of true scientific study or peer-reviewed publication. This type of evidence is easy to gather because it requires no formal study, no scientific protocols, and no peer review. The problem with knee arthritis treatments today is that there is far too much anecdotal evidence being used in place of true scientific evidence.

Individual *patient testimonies* are not given credence when it comes to scientific proof of efficacy. It seems that patient testimonies are great marketing tools, but when deciding on a medical treatment, I urge you to consider them worthless. I suggest caution when using only the experience of one neighbor, family member, or friend when deciding how to treat your knee pain.

Patients are often misled by anecdotal evidence and patient testimonies and are instead led to believe that a treatment is so cutting edge that large studies have not been done. This is rarely true, and those treatments might require cash payments because insurance companies won't cover treatments that are unproven. When cash payments are taken for knee arthritis treatments that are not backed by a reasonable level of scientific evidence or administered as part of a well-designed scientific study, its often ethically inappropriate and false advertising.

A final reason to consider treatments backed by science rather than anecdote or testimony is that safety is often part of the scientific evaluation. A treatment that is proven to be safe is far more valuable than one that "appears" safe but has not been properly studied.

## The Placebo Effect

The *placebo effect* is an incompletely understood, but real and accepted phenomenon that occurs in the human body. This effect occurs when only the idea of a treatment has the proposed effect of the treatment. Think of taking a pill that patients are told is a new pain medication; yet, (unknown to those taking it) that pill is made only of sugar. If the subjects BELIEVE it is a pain pill, a percentage of patients taking that sugar pill will report less pain, even though pain should not decrease in response to low-dose sugar ingestion alone. The placebo effect is a fascinating example of the power of the human brain.

This is an important concept to understand because many treatments offered for arthritis likely function through the placebo effect. Placebos are critical in scientific research because treatments being tested are often compared to a placebo treatment in order to determine whether the intended treatment effect is physiologic or a product of the placebo effect. Not every available treatment marketed for knee osteoarthritis has been studied properly in this manner.

## How to Use This Book

It is important to note that this book is about treatments for knee *osteoarthritis*. Chapter 2 talks about the kinds of arthritis in the knee and different types may have specific recommendations. Osteoarthritis is by far the most common. For simplicity going forward, the terms osteoarthritis and arthritis will be used interchangeably.

I have intentionally avoided an in-depth discussion of the scientific papers behind the treatment options listed to make the book more readable. There are, however, some references in this book that are necessary to give other authors and organizations credit for their work.

First-line treatments are identified clearly. Treatment programs for knee arthritis should start with some combination of these. Second-line and third-line treatments should be considered if first-line are not effective or not medically advised.

This book is not a substitute for individualized medical care. It is a reference to give you a background to discuss this information with your personal medical professional(s). Every medical practitioner has different training backgrounds, sources of information, and patient care experiences. Every patient has different needs, beliefs, and medical conditions.

## Secrets of Knee Arthritis Treatments

One of the most important themes in this book is that there are no secrets. Anyone who tells you that he has a secret fix, elixir, or other treatment to cure your arthritis is selling you snake oil. When we talk about treating osteoarthritis non-operatively, we are not actually treating arthritis, but rather, the SYMPTOMS. This is an important concept to understand. I wish I could deliver a non-surgical product that definitively cured pain or reversed the effects of osteoarthritis. No such treatment currently exists; but, someday, we may have that capability.

## Conflicts of Interest

The author and publisher of this book have no conflicts of interest or paid relationships with medical device companies, drug companies, or any other financial incentives that would cause us to recommend one treatment over another. Any potential conflicts of interest that arise after the publication date of this book are disclosed on www.orthoskool.com.

## Chapter 1 Review

- There is a lot of information out there. Obtaining the RIGHT information is critical to understanding options to treat knee pain.

- Not all scientific papers and medical claims are equal.

- Beware of treatments that are backed by only anecdotal evidence and patient testimony.

- Treatments backed by science are safer and more efficacious than those with no formal study.

- This book should be used for information purposes, but you should discuss the best treatments for YOU with a licensed medical practitioner.

Chapter Two

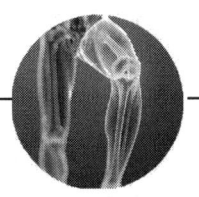

# The Basics of Knee Arthritis

If you have *chronic* knee pain, you probably remember a time when you were pain-free. As children and teenagers, most of us were active and not limited by joint pain. Some describe the feeling of their youth as "being invincible". We could run, jump, skip, pivot, and dance for hours without pain. Our knees were no different than our earlobes in that that it was a body part and not a pain generator. If you have knee pain from arthritis, it's possible that you are aware of your knee joint every day, maybe with every step.
In this chapter, I define the normal anatomy of the knee and the condition of arthritis. I also describe how the invincible knee can become the burdensome knee. With these building blocks in place, we will have .the background to discuss treatment options in upcoming chapters

## Knee Anatomy – The Invincible Knee Before Arthritis

We are going to stick to the basics, but first, you should learn about the anatomy of the normal knee before we move on to what can go wrong.

The knee is medically known as a *hinge joint*: a joint that primarily bends and straightens in one plane of motion. The knee joint consists of **three bones** which play important roles in its form and function (Figure 2-1). The *fibula* is a close-by fourth bone that supports the knee joint, the lower leg, and the ankle joint, but does not play a key role in knee arthritis.

The three major bones are:
1. *Femur*: Your thigh bone. The longest bone in the body, extending from your hip joint to your knee joint

2. *Tibia*: Your shin bone, which extends from the knee to the ankle.
3. *Patella*: Your kneecap. This bone glides up and down in a groove on the femur bone as your knee bends and straightens.

The normal knee has two types of *cartilage* in it (Figure 2-1). *Cartilage* is typically soft and protects bones from rubbing together. All joints have cartilage in them. The types of cartilage in the knee include:

1. *Articular cartilage* (also called surface cartilage): This is a smooth, slick surface that covers the end of the femur, tibia, and backside of the patella. Think of this as a coating over the bones that is typically < 3 mm thick. In a healthy knee, articular cartilage allows the joint surfaces to glide past each other with minimal friction.
2. *Meniscus* (plural = *menisci)*: These are two c-shaped cartilage wedges that serve as shock absorbers in the knee joint. They protect the articular cartilage as well as the underlying bone from damage.

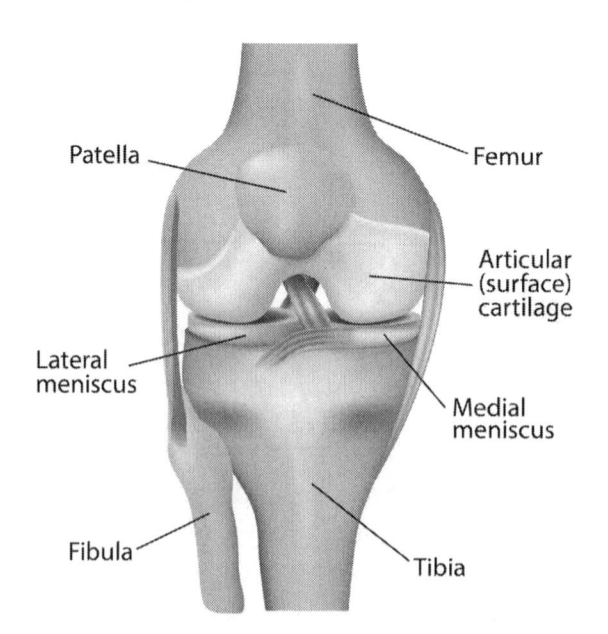

**Figure 2-1**: Bones and cartilage that make up the knee joint.

The bones that make up the knee joint are held together by soft tissues. Your knee has several soft (but strong) tissue structures that serve two purposes: to support your knee, and to assist with bending/straightening. *Ligaments* connect two bones together. They are *static* supporting structures because they stay in one place and resist stretching and movement. *Tendons* connect muscles to bone. We call them *dynamic* supporting structures because the muscles contract to apply tension around the joints. The ligaments and tendons within the knee joint are shown in Figure 2-2.

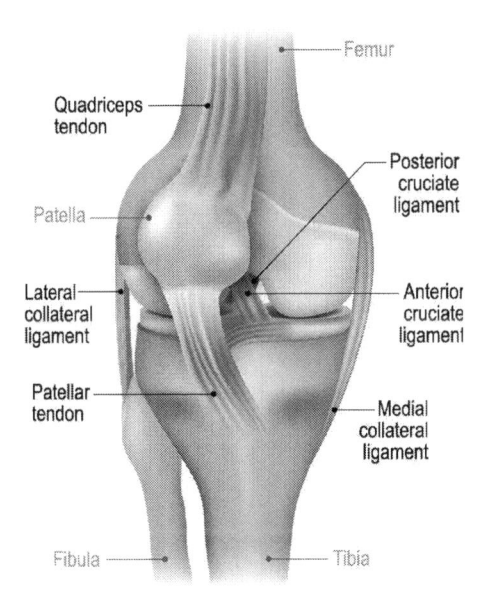

**Figure 2-2**: Supporting soft tissue structures in the knee joint include ligaments and tendons.

There are three *compartments* in the knee. Compartments are areas of the knee where cartilage covering two bones *articulate* (the medical term for "rub together"). There are three distinct parts of the knee where cartilage-covered bones articulate:

1. *Medial compartment*: *medial* means "toward the midline of the body", this compartment is found in the inner side of the knee.
2. *Lateral compartment*: *lateral* means "away from the midline of the body", this compartment is found in the outer part of the knee

3. *Patellofemoral compartment*: this is the compartment where the *patella* glides up and down a groove in the femur called the *trochlea*. There is cartilage both on the backside of the *patella* and in the *trochlea*.

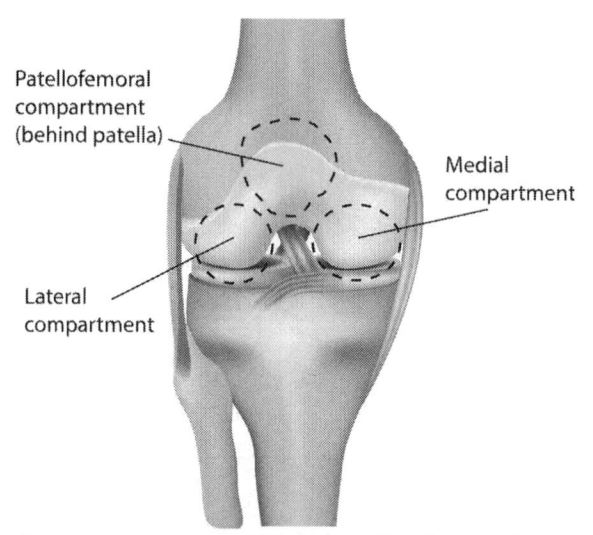

**Figure 2-3**: The three compartments of the knee joint. The patella has been removed for better visualization. These are areas where cartilage surfaces rub together.

## Knee Arthritis – The Burdensome Knee

The word "arthritis" originates from two Greek words – *arthron*, meaning "joint" and *itis*, a medical suffix attached to any medical condition characterized by inflammation. When you combine these two words, you get a new word, *arthr-itis*, or "inflamed joint". Similar examples include *col-itis* (inflamed colon) and *bronch-itis* (inflamed bronchi).

*Inflammation* of the knee joint is often associated with cartilage wear. Cartilage wear has become synonymous with arthritis. Cartilage wear occurs when the few millimeters of cartilage covering the ends of the bone deteriorates, exposing the bone underneath. When a person has significant inflammation and cartilage wear, pain is the common result. Figure 2-4 compares the normal knee to the arthritic knee.

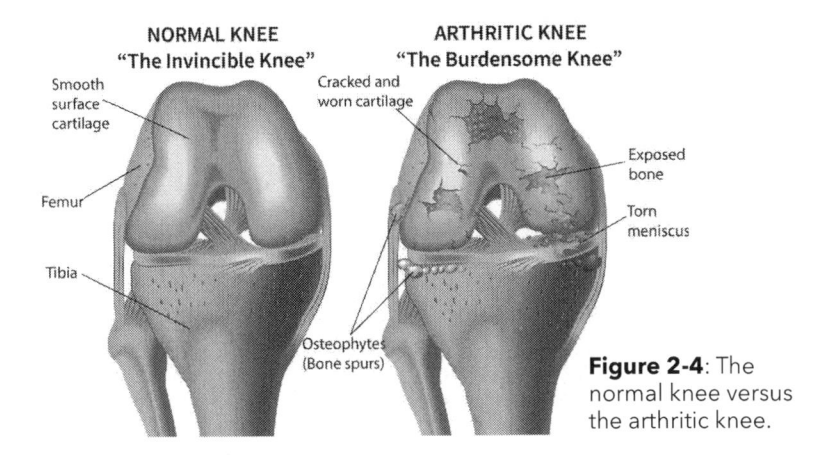

**Figure 2-4**: The normal knee versus the arthritic knee.

## How Arthritis is Diagnosed

The definitive test to diagnose arthritis is x-ray. Physicians use several criteria to diagnose arthritis with x-ray, but the two most common are:

1. *Cartilage space narrowing*: Bone always shows up on an x-ray and cartilage does not – it is transparent on x-ray. A classic x-ray sign of cartilage wear is a narrowing of the transparent space where the cartilage used to be.

2. *Osteophytes*: As a protective mechanism during cartilage wear, outcroppings of bone and/or cartilage form at the edge of the knee joint. These are commonly called "bone spurs". Bone spurs are another telltale x-ray sign of cartilage wear.

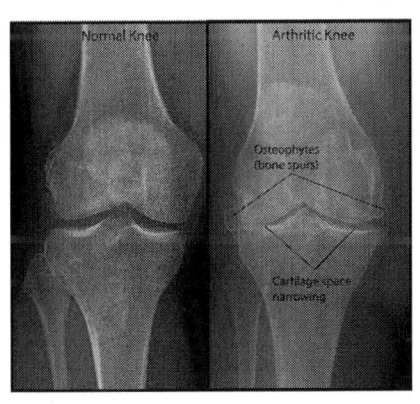

**Figure 2-5**: A normal knee x-ray compared to the arthritic knee x-ray. Note the cartilage space narrowing and osteophytes in the arthritic knee.

Using x-ray, your doctor can rate the severity of your arthritis.

- If you have *mild arthritis*, you will have minimal cartilage space narrowing.
- If you have *moderate arthritis*, at least 50 percent of your available cartilage space will be gone while some osteophytes may be present.
- If you have *severe arthritis*, in at least one area of your knee, there will be full-thickness loss of cartilage, a condition known as *bone-on-bone arthritis*.

It is important to note that advanced imaging such as CT scan and MRI are typically not needed if arthritis is seen on x-ray. These advanced studies are only helpful if the diagnosis is in doubt after the x-ray.

## Common Misconceptions about Arthritis

Some people think arthritis is a material that forms in the knee. Arthritis is a medical condition, not a substance. You cannot scrape away, remove, or clean out inflammation and cartilage wear. It is less like the tartar that builds up on your teeth than it is like the wear on your car tires in areas where the tread is gone.

Perhaps the confusion is because when we look at an x-ray, we can see those bone spurs (osteophytes) that form in response to arthritis. However, you should know that these bone spurs are just a feature or sign of arthritis and not the arthritis itself. Removal of this feature does not cure the disease.

Regarding arthritis features, let us quickly identify some other features that often present with arthritis (although not always). One feature is *pain*. Arthritis-related pain is complicated. For reasons that the medical community does not fully understand, arthritis does not always result in pain. In addition, the severity of arthritis as seen on an x-ray is not directly proportional to the amount of pain you may experience. In other words, we cannot tell how much pain you are having just by looking at your x-ray. Some patients with mild arthritis may have severe pain, while others with severe arthritis may not have pain at all.

Another optional arthritis feature is *deformity*. In orthopedic terms, *deformity* simply means angulation of the joint. Some patients with knee arthritis may become bow-legged (*varus* deformity). This occurs when the cartilage on the *medial* compartment wears out faster than the lateral compartment. Other patients may become knock-kneed (*valgus* deformity), where the lateral compartment wears out first.

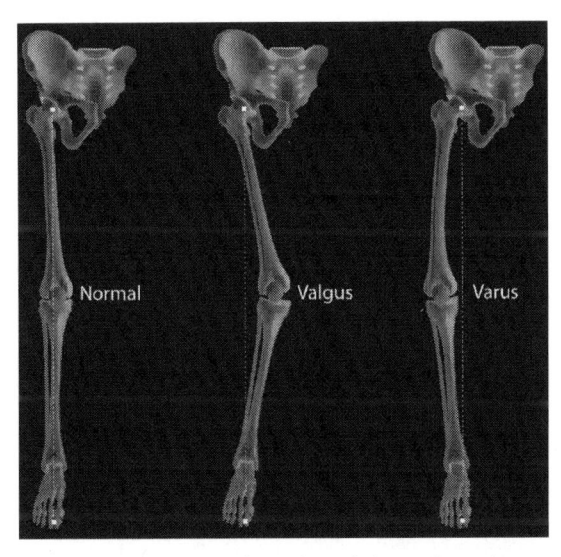

**Figure 2-6:** Normal knee alignment, valgus (knock-kneed), and varus (bow-legged) deformities of the knee.

## Types of Knee Arthritis

There are three major types of knee arthritis. Each type has a unique underlying cause but produces a similar painful condition.

### Osteoarthritis

The first is *osteoarthritis*. This is by far the most common type, and the focus of this book. It is called "wear and tear" arthritis because it often has no identifiable cause and is more prevalent with age. *Osteoarthritis* is commonly confused with *osteoporosis*; however, they are not the same. *Osteoporosis* is a problem within the structure of a bone that results in decreased bone density, which then causes bones to fracture easily.

## Inflammatory arthritis

*Inflammatory arthritis* describes a group of diseases where excess inflammation occurs in the joints for unknown reasons, and cartilage wear follows.

*Rheumatoid arthritis* is the most common type of inflammatory arthritis. This is an *autoimmune* disorder, where the body's immune system is overactive and works against joint surfaces to break down otherwise healthy cartilage and bone.

Most people with inflammatory arthritis have seen a rheumatologist and are on special medications to treat their systemic condition. This book does not cover treatments for inflammatory arthritis.

## Post-traumatic arthritis

The third is *post-traumatic arthritis*. This occurs when a trauma such as a fracture occurs within the joint surface leading to permanent damage. When the cartilage sustains significant damage, it may do well for a period; however, over the course of months or years, worsening arthritis develops. Treatments are the same as for osteoarthritis, so this treatments in this book are relevant for post-traumatic conditions.

# What Causes Osteoarthritis?

This question comes up frequently. It is easier to understand why cartilage wear occurs with inflammatory and post-traumatic arthritis. However, osteoarthritis is complex and *multifactorial*, which means that there are several factors that contribute to it. There are *inherent* (things you can't change) and *modifiable* (things you can change) risk factors for the development of osteoarthritis (Table 2-1):

## Inherent Risk Factors – things you cannot change

- Genetic makeup: Your genes play a large role in osteoarthritis, but their exact role is not fully understood. It is not as simple as skin color or height, which can often be predicted based on your parents. Multiple genes play a role, and the interactions and expression of those genes are under current investigation.

**Table 2-1:** Inherent and modifiable risk factors for osteoarthritis

| Inherent Risk Factors | Modifiable |
|---|---|
| Genetic makeup | Excess body mass |
| Gender | Sport/occupation stresses |
| Age | |
| Minor injury | |
| Luck | |

- Gender: Osteoarthritis is more common and more severe in women than men.
- Age: There is a clear correlation with age and prevalence of osteoarthritis.
- Injury: When a patient has a prior major injury such as a fracture within the knee joint or a ligament injury, we classify subsequent arthritis as post-traumatic. Patients may not recall a time long ago when they had a minor twisting injury to their knee that hurt for a few days and resolved without ever seeing a doctor. We believe that some of these seemingly minor injuries can result in osteoarthritis much later in life.
- Luck: Because there are so many potential causes of osteoarthritis and much of this we still do not understand, we tell patients that there is some luck involved.

## Modifiable Risk Factors—things you can change

- Excess body mass: Excess body weight can be a sensitive subject, but it is clearly linked to osteoarthritis. Obesity has reached pandemic status worldwide. Body mass affects knee arthritis in two ways. The first is intuitive: increased weight (or load) on cartilage surfaces increases the rate of wear. The second is less intuitive (and maybe more important): excess fat tissue secretes molecules in the body that increase inflammation and are thought to cause cartilage surfaces to break down. When these two mechanisms are working together, they cause the cartilage in your knees to wear at a rate higher than they would if you were at your ideal body weight. See "Calculation of Body Mass Index" below to figure out your ideal body weight.

- Sport and occupation stress: It may seem intuitive that more weight-bearing activities and stress on the knee joint would cause more wear. This is the common historical teaching of medical providers. Research has not proven this to be definitively true. Running, for example, is considered one of the biggest stressors on the knee joint, yet several studies have shown that runners do not have an increased risk of knee arthritis. There is also a theory that exercise strengthens bones and joints and therefore provides a protective effect against cartilage wear, which may counteract wear. Here is what I tell my patients: avoid running, sports, and activities that cause knee pain because if it's causing pain, it's probably causing damage; but if you can run marathons without pain in your knees, it's probably fine to continue.

## The Progression of Knee Osteoarthritis

The natural history of knee arthritis, regardless of the type or cause, involves progression over time. Symptoms include pain and inflammation. In addition, the inability to exercise and walk long distances tends to worsen. The progression of knee osteoarthritis is often in a variable stepwise fashion, meaning it does not increase at a constant rate, but gets better, then worse, then better, then worse, etc.

Figure 2-7 shows an example of the stepwise progression of pain over time. Note the areas labeled *"flare"*. It is common for patients to show up at a doctor's office with a bout of severe pain in a knee that has been only mildly symptomatic in the past, only to find that x-rays show the *chronic* condition of arthritis may have been there for months or years. The period of flare tends to last days or weeks, but usually improves, especially after utilizing some of the treatments listed in Chapter 3.

> **Calculation of Body Mass Index**
>
> Search the Internet for "body mass index calculator." Several will come up, and any will do the job. Enter your height and weight when prompted. Calculate your *body mass index* (BMI). Once you have calculated this, compare your BMI to the numbers below as published by the Centers for Disease Control:
>
> Underweight <18.5
> Healthy Range 18.5 – 24.9
> Overweight 25.0 – 29.9
> Obese ≥30.0
>
> Obese Class I: 30 – 34.9
> Obese Class II: 35 – 39.9
> Obese Class III: ≥40 (also called "extreme" or "severe" obesity)
>
> If your BMI is >30, you should strongly consider weight loss. If your BMI is >35, then you have a serious health condition that needs immediate attention. If your BMI is over forty, you should not be considering any elective surgical procedure until you have lost weight. This is a general guideline and may not apply to muscular individuals who are lean.

X-rays also tend to worsen with time. Progressive cartilage space narrowing is the most common finding on an x-ray, and we will often see enlarging osteophytes and increasing deformity (more varus or valgus deformity).

The condition of arthritis encompasses a spectrum of symptoms where some patients may not be able to run but can perform all other activities pain-free. Another patient may have trouble standing, walking, or sleeping at night. On the severe end, symptoms can be debilitating and require a walker or wheelchair.

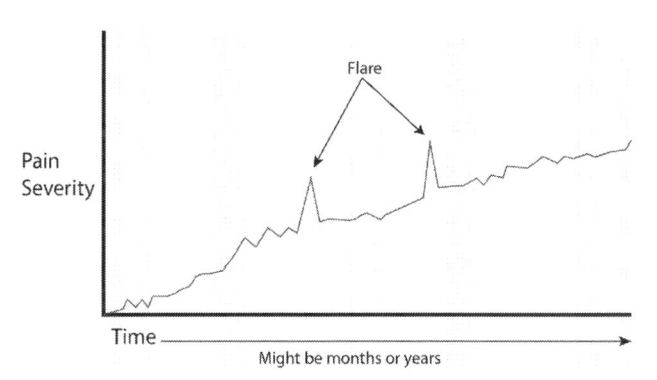

**Figure 2-7:** An example of the stepwise and variable progression of arthritis symptoms over time. The severity of pain over time will be different for every knee. Note the areas of worsening and improvement, with severe worsening known as "flare".

## Chapter 2 Review

- Arthritis = joint inflammation + cartilage wear.
- Arthritis is not a substance in your knee, it is a condition.
- Bone spurs are a result of arthritis and a sign we see on x-ray. They are not the cause of pain and are not the underlying problem.
- There are three main types of arthritis:
- Osteoarthritis
- Inflammatory arthritis
- Post-traumatic arthritis
- The cause of osteoarthritis is *multifactorial*, with many factors that you cannot control.
- Body mass index is important in determining your risk for arthritis and your risk for overall health problems.
- Arthritis tends to progress over time with respect to symptoms and x-ray findings, respectively.
- A "flare" of arthritis is a dramatic acute worsening of symptoms that lasts from days to weeks but usually improves.
- Arthritis encompasses a spectrum of diseases; symptoms can range from mild discomfort to severe and debilitating pain.

Chapter Three

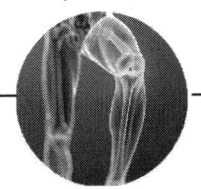

# Lifestyle Changes

Some of the most effective ways to treat knee arthritis do not involve medications, injections, or surgery. Whether you are looking for non-operative treatments or end up having surgery, what follows in this chapter is important for your health and overall outcome.

As a society, we have learned to appreciate quick fixes. Patients are often disappointed to learn that there is no pill, injection, or another quick fix currently available to cure knee arthritis. Most treatments come at the price of time and effort, and nobody can do it for you. I urge you to take the recommendations in this chapter seriously if you are serious about alleviating knee pain without surgery.

## Your Primary Care Provider

Your general health is the foundation from which all abnormal conditions arise. By managing your overall health, you are managing your knee arthritis. To do this effectively, you should have an established *primary care provider* (PCP). This is an easy, no-risk recommendation for every adult. If you don't have one, find one. This could be a doctor, nurse practitioner, or physician assistant. Medical specialties that serve in the primary care provider role for adults include family practice, internal medicine, geriatrics, and in some cases gynecology/obstetrics. PCPs are a wonderful, caring group of medical providers that have a broad range of knowledge. If you develop a relationship with one, they get to know you and your medical history, which increases the quality of care. Most of the treatments in this book are offered by PCPs, and they will help you find the best specialist if your condition is outside of their area of expertise.

> ## Weight Loss
>
> **Recommendation:** YES – first-line treatment. Weight loss is strongly recommended for anyone with a BMI >30.
>
> **Risk**: Low

Weight loss affects your knee in two ways. First, it decreases knee pain. There are multiple studies that have shown this. In some cases, weight loss may negate the need for surgery. Second, weight loss decreases the rate of cartilage wear in an arthritic knee. It is one of the only known risk factors for the advancement of arthritis that we can modify.

Weight loss also has substantial effects on your overall health. Having excess *adipose tissue* (fat tissue) causes a state of inflammation that affects every system in the body. Further, if you end up needing a joint replacement, the surgery will be safer, and you will be more satisfied with the outcome in a lower weight class. How much should you lose? There is no right answer to this. Any weight loss is better than nothing, and the closer you are to ideal BMI, the better.

Return to Chapter Two and read how to calculate your BMI if you have not done it yet. If you have knee pain or arthritis, and your BMI is >30, try to lose weight loss. There is no downside to weight loss other than the time, effort, and commitment that goes into it. There is no other treatment available in this book (or on the planet) that has the potential to decrease pain, decrease the rate of arthritis wear, potentially help you avoid surgery, and improve your overall health and happiness like weight loss.

Weight loss can be life-changing for anyone, with or without knee pain. In order to accomplish something that is life-changing, you will have to make significant changes in life. "How?" you may ask. That question is the basis of a weight-loss industry worth over $70 billion in the United States alone. There is no single right answer. It doesn't matter if you count calories, weigh your food, avoid carbohydrates, start a new exercise program, join a gym, buy a book, or pay money to undertake one of the so-called "fad" diets with catchy and well-known names. The simple fact is that you need to commit to a plan and expect it to require persistent work. It will not be easy, but you also don't have to be perfect. You just need to make lasting changes that over time will result in weight loss. Seek help, find support, and YOU CAN DO THIS!

> ### Low-Impact Aerobic Exercise
>
> **Recommendation:** YES–first-line treatment. Aim for 20-60 minutes of low-impact, moderate-intensity aerobic exercise three days per week.
>
> **Risk**: Low–but check with your primary care doctor to ensure this is safe for you. Avoid activities that aggravate knee pain.

This is the type of exercise that elevates your heart rate and breathing for sustained periods of time. This type of exercise should be a cornerstone of health for most adults. Take on a low-impact exercise program only if it can be done with minimal or no pain. Knee osteoarthritis generally responds well to low-impact exercise, even for those with severe cartilage wear. Patients with either severe arthritis or severe symptoms may have to work hard to find an activity that they can do without significant pain. It may take some trial and error to find what works for you.

Patients are sometimes concerned that moving an arthritic joint will advance the cartilage wear. This seems logical, but the available studies show that active adults have less knee pain than adults with equivalent arthritis on x-ray but are sedentary. The body wants to move, and joints that move tend to hurt less.

In 2018, the U.S. Department of Health and Human Services published the Physical Activity Guidelines for Americans, 2nd edition.[1] Their recommendations state that exercise should include at least 150 minutes of moderate-intensity, or 75 minutes of vigorous-intensity aerobic physical activity each week, or some mixture of the two. Those who follow these recommendations will have an overall improvement in health, sleep, happiness and decrease the risk of developing chronic medical conditions.

**Land-based** low-impact activities include outdoor or indoor cycling, elliptical trainer, rowing, cross-country skiing, and strength-based yoga. I have a personal bias toward cycling and believe that riding a bike with low to moderate sustained resistance (enough to cause thigh muscle fatigue) is particularly beneficial for patients with knee pain. I prefer a traditional upright stationary or outdoor bike for those who can tolerate it, but a recumbent bicycle is just fine for those who cannot. Walking outdoors or on a treadmill is considered a moderate-impact activity as it puts a more repetitive impact on the joints than others listed above.

**Water-based** (pool) low-impact exercises including swimming, water aerobics, water walking, water jogging, or using water weights are all excellent options for patients with arthritis because the buoyancy of the water reduces pressure on the joints. The water also provides resistance to movement.

If the above suggestions do not work with you, or you feel you need more guidance, check with a licensed physical therapist or a personal trainer at your local gym to find a low-impact routine that fits your needs.

> ### High-Impact Exercise
>
> **Recommendation:** NO—avoid high-impact exercise if you have existing knee arthritis or knee pain.
>
> **Risk**: Moderate to High—you risk advancing cartilage wear, pain, and swelling.

If you have knee arthritis or knee pain, you should avoid high-impact activities. These include activities such as running, basketball, soccer, gymnastics, box jumps, high-intensity interval training, or any other activity that puts sudden, forceful, or jarring loads on the knees.

For decades, orthopedic surgeons have recommended against distance running for fear that joints will wear more quickly. Interestingly, studies show a low incidence of knee and hip arthritis in marathon runners. I don't believe that running alone CAUSES cartilage wear. If you have no pain, high-impact exercise activities can be safe, fun, and good for your cardiovascular health. If you have pain, you might be doing damage, so you should look for a low-impact aerobic activity.

> ### How can I lose weight when my knee hurts? I can't exercise!
>
> If you truly cannot exercise due to knee pain, you absolutely can still lose weight. One of the most common misconceptions in weight loss is that patients believe they cannot lose weight without burning more calories. It turns out that diet is far more important than exercise when it comes to weight loss. This information is well distributed in both scientific journals and in mainstream media, but as a society, we have missed the message and, in some cases, we don't want to believe it. Both diet and exercise can help, but of the two, diet is more important.

> ## Mental Health Maintenance
>
> **Recommendation:** YES–first-line treatment. All patients should pay close attention to their mental health.
>
> **Risk**: Low

The power of the human brain is astounding. It controls so much more of our health than we give it credit for. Research shows a link between pain and mental health conditions. In particular, numerous anxiety and depression studies show a connection with pain. In addition, those with mental health disorders have more difficulty coping with health conditions and decisions. It makes sense to connect mental health and pain because our thoughts and pain are both driven by the nervous system. This is a fascinating field of science that begs the question of cause and effect: which came first, the mental health disorder or the pain?

For patients with chronic pain, strongly consider a mental health evaluation. Your primary care doctor is equipped to screen for this and is a great place to start. There are many treatment options for mental health disorders that have a secondary benefit of decreasing chronic pain. Treatments may include medications, behavioral therapy, therapy with a mental health professional, and mindfulness exercises.

The term *mindfulness* describes a state of living whereby we guide ourselves to live in the moment. The idea is that we gain control over our thoughts, feelings, and emotions. Mindfulness practices have been around for centuries, but over the last decade, we have seen a rise in the number studies showing benefits, and a surge in the number of Americans who utilize mindfulness in their daily lives. See the Appendix for resources on mindfulness and meditation.

## Chapter 3 Review

- The recommended lifestyle changes listed are all considered first-line treatments for knee osteoarthritis.
- Patients who take charge of education and treatment options for their own medical conditions have better outcomes.
- Weight loss is one of the most important ways to treat and prevent knee arthritis. Not only does it decrease knee pain, but it is also one of the only known modifiable risk factors for future wear of cartilage.
- Low-impact exercise is important for your overall health, and it can decrease your knee pain in the presence of arthritis.
- Avoid high-impact exercise if you have knee pain or existing knee arthritis.
- You can lose weight without exercise. Diet is more important than exercise in the weight loss game.

Chapter Four

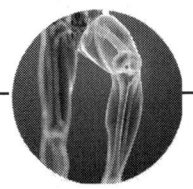

# Physical Therapy and Complementary Therapies

Physical and complementary therapies are widely used and accepted treatments for knee arthritis. These are therapies that manipulate tissues on the outside of the body to help with conditions inside the body. They typically do not involve chemicals, medications, or injections, and as a class of treatments are considered safe. Let's go through the most common types and discuss the efficacy of each.

> ### Formal Physical Therapy (PT)
> **Recommendation:** YES—first-line treatment. PT is worth trying for any patient with existing knee arthritis or knee pain.
>
> **Risk**: Low

When we talk about formal, supervised physical therapy, it is important to note that this is different from a low-impact exercise program or resistance training that you do on your own. Physical therapists know how to evaluate patients for weaknesses and strengths, how to stretch and manipulate soft tissues, and they know how to target muscle groups for specific conditions. Technique and timing are extremely important in rehabilitation, and you need a coach. Further, working with a physical therapist can give you some accountability to follow a program and he can provide objective measures of progress.

Multiple studies have shown that strengthening muscle groups in the legs can improve both strength and function in the presence of arthritis. It often takes a minimum of six weeks of dedicated work to note improvement, and up to a year to see maximum improvement if muscular weakness and deconditioning are contributing to knee pain. The exercises should be done a minimum of three days per week for four to six weeks to see a difference in symptoms. Going to a therapist once or twice is not expected to relieve your problem. Use your therapy sessions as coaching sessions and progress checks, but the real work happens when you are on your own in between sessions. If you approach it this way, you increase your chance of achieving good results.

> ### Strength Training on Your Own
>
> **Recommendation:** YES–first-line treatment. Do this only after you receive training on how to do the exercises correctly.
>
> **Risk**: Low, if exercises are performed correctly

Some patients have the strength training experience to do effective work on their own. Remember that form and technique are CRITICAL, so I stand by my recommendation for formal PT. Consider at least one or two sessions with a licensed therapist or experienced trainer before you create your own program. As a practicing orthopedic surgeon, I have sought the advice of physical therapists for my own musculoskeletal ailments and found them invaluable. You should do the same.

If you insist on being your own strength coach, focus on the specific muscle groups listed below. Some of my favorite exercises are in the Appendix. Try a strengthening program for three or more days per week. It often takes four to six weeks to see a difference, but many patients need an ongoing maintenance program to fend off pain. Avoid any exercises that cause knee pain.

- Quadriceps: this group is the most important stabilizer of the knee joint. If you have arthritis behind the patella (patellofemoral joint), avoid loaded knee extensions.

- Hamstrings: The hamstrings are also an important dynamic stabilizer of the knee joint.
- Hip flexors, hip abductors, and calf muscles: the muscles above and below the knee joint certainly have an effect on knee stability and dynamics.

> ### Stretching on Your Own
>
> **Recommendation:** YES–first-line treatment. Do this after you receive training on how to stretch correctly
>
> **Risk**: Low, if stretching is performed correctly

Some patients, especially those with milder arthritis, may benefit from gentle stretching of the muscles and tendons around the knee. I'll repeat my ongoing recommendation to have your stretching program supervised by a physical therapist to ensure proper technique and intensity. As with strengthening programs, it may take six weeks to see a difference.

Muscle groups to focus on are similar to those that benefit from strengthening include quadriceps, hamstrings, hip flexors, calf muscles, and iliotibial band. Some of my favorite stretches are shown in the Appendix.

> ### Knee Stretching and Strengthening Rules
>
> - Form and technique are critical
> - Perform exercises least three days per week
> - Be consistent: set up a routine and stick to it
> - Be patient: it may take six weeks to see a difference

> ### Electrotherapeutic Modalities
>
> **Recommendation:** YES–second-line treatment. It must be supervised by a therapist. Note that high-level scientific evidence for efficacy is lacking.
>
> **Risk**: Low, if administered by a professional

Electrical stimulation of muscles and nerves by placing electrodes on the skin has had reported therapeutic benefits in different parts of the body. The idea is that if we stimulate muscles to contract it can aid in growth and strength. There is also a theory that electrical impulses stimulate the body to address pain via native pain regulators. Several forms of stimulation exist including transcutaneous electrical nerve stimulation (TENS), neuromuscular electrical stimulation (NMES), interferential current (IFC), pulsed electrical stimulation (PES), and others.

This type of therapy has been difficult to study because of the different modalities and intensities of stimulation available. Overall the scientific data is quite mixed on whether it is effective for treating knee pain from arthritis. There is not an overwhelming consensus as to whether these therapies work or do not work.

Find a physical therapist that you trust. If they use one of these modalities in their practice, I see little harm and potentially some benefit.

---

### Massage Therapy

**Recommendation:** YES—second-line treatment. It's worth trying but only supported by low-level scientific evidence.

**Risk:** Low, but consider the monetary cost versus effect

---

Massage therapy has been shown to provide some patients with temporary relief of knee pain from osteoarthritis. The studies that show this are generally of low quality, and those that show benefit tend to demonstrate a short duration of pain relief. There is certainly a component of soft tissue inflammation around the knee in patients with knee arthritis, so this could address that component. I believe this is a low-risk and worthwhile treatment option and worth trying with a licensed massage therapist, with the understanding that it's more likely to provide short-term relief than long-lasting relief.

## Heat and Cold Therapy

**Recommendation:** YES–first-line treatment. You have the tools for this at home already.

**Risk**: Low

Heat and cold therapy have been used for years to relieve arthritis pain. Both are worth trying, and both do not work in all patients.

For heat, use a shower, bath, hot tub, or heating pad BEFORE exercise or activity. This can loosen up the joint and make it feel more mobile. Never place a heating pad directly on the skin as I've seen them burn more than one patient.

For cold therapy, try either ice packs or a commercially available ice machine. Always ice AFTER, not before, physical activity. Some patients use bags of frozen vegetables and I think they work well. Never place ice bags directly on the skin—put a towel or other material between the bag and the skin to avoid burns. 20-30 minutes on the knee up to three times per day may provide some relief from pain and swelling.

## Acupuncture

**Recommendation:** NO–due to the lack of well-designed studies showing efficacy.

**Risk**: Low

Acupuncture is a form of traditional Chinese medicine that involves the insertion of tiny needles into the skin at targeted points on the body that is proposed to affect pain and even physiologic processes in some cases. From a scientific standpoint, several studies have looked at whether acupuncture effectively treats arthritis pain. The overall quality of the available studies is low, and the results are mixed. The studies showing the greatest effect compared acupuncture to no treatment, which brings into question the placebo effect. It should be noted that the American Academy of Orthopaedic Surgeons (AAOS) 2013 guidelines state a strong recommendation against the use of acupuncture for knee arthritis pain based on lack of efficacy.[2] The American College of Rheumatology conditionally recommends acupuncture only in the circumstance that moderate to severe arthritis is present and the patient is unwilling or unable to undergo knee replacement.[3]

Some patients like the idea that this treatment moves outside of the theories of Western medicine. If this fits your beliefs and you can afford the cost, this risk of this treatment is low. It's reasonable to expect that any symptomatic relief would be temporary, and acupuncture will not serve as a long-term solution for most patients.

---

**Therapeutic Ultrasound**

**Recommendation:** NO–due to lack of quality scientific data

**Risk**: Low

---

Ultrasound is used in medicine primarily as an imaging technique but has been studied as a therapeutic measure in osteoarthritis. The available studies have unimpressive results. While this is a low-risk option, it's hard to make an argument to pursue this as a legitimate treatment.

---

**Cupping and Laser Therapy**

**Recommendation:** NO–due to lack of quality scientific data

**Risk**: Low

---

Cupping and laser therapy are trendy options for knee arthritis and pain in general. It is difficult to recommend either based on the paucity of available research. It has been interesting to see a surge in cupping after the most decorated Olympian of all-time showed up with cupping marks on his body at the 2016 Olympic Games. Well-designed, quality studies are lacking for both cupping and laser therapy. My suggestion is to not spend money on these treatments until better data is available.

## Chapter 4 Review

- Formal physical therapy, strength training, and gentle stretching are all recommended as options in treating knee osteoarthritis pain

- Electrotherapeutic modalities, massage therapy, and heat/cold therapy may have some pain benefits and are generally safe, but scientific evidence behind them is not strong

- Acupuncture has poor scientific evidence as a long-term treatment for arthritis pain, but some select patients may benefit. Cost of treatments versus effect should be considered.

- Therapeutic ultrasound, cupping therapy, and laser therapy are not recommended.

Chapter Five

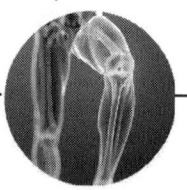

# Injections

Medications injected into the knee joint have become a staple of treatment for knee arthritis. Let's be clear that nothing we currently have available for knee injections regrows cartilage or protects cartilage from future wear. The goal of these injections is to improve symptoms, not modify the structures within the knee joint.

A note of caution with injections for those planning knee surgery. Any injection into a joint has the risk of introducing bacteria into the joint space. There is some data that shows an increased risk of infection with knee replacement surgery when an injection has been given within <u>three months</u> of the surgery date. This recommendation used to exist only for cortisone injections, but studies have shown a risk with other types of injections as well. The risk seems to be time-dependent, with closer proximity increasing the odds of infection. Avoid ANY needles in the knee if surgery is planned within three months.

---

### Cortisone Injections

**Recommendation:** YES–first-line treatment. Most patients get some symptomatic relief, but the duration is variable.

**Risk**: Low to moderate (see below for a description of risks)

---

Most people know these as *cortisone* injections, but they are commonly called *steroid* or *corticosteroid* injections. All three names are synonymous. Corticosteroids have been used in many disciplines of medicine since the 1950s, and they are also produced naturally in the body. Cortisone suppresses some inflammatory enzymes which results in less pain, less inflammation, and less swelling in the knee joint.

Cortisone injections are one of the most widely administered treatments for knee arthritis. Despite the widespread use, the quality of the research behind their efficacy is relatively low. I think most medical practitioners and patients agree that for short-term relief, this is a reasonable option that is readily available and safe.

There are many types of cortisone that are used for this application. My preference is triamcinolone, but this is admittedly based on limited scientific data and more on experience. There is also no good data that tells us how much to give and how often it should be given.

I tell my patients that most receiving cortisone will get some relief, though it may not offer complete resolution of symptoms. The duration of relief is typically less than three months. I believe one of the main reasons to give a steroid injection is to allow for enough pain relief to do physical therapy and low-impact exercise. These injections are particularly effective in the case of an osteoarthritis flare (see Chapter Two). I have also seen cases where a single injection gives long-term relief.

There are a few warnings to be aware of with steroid injections, but I don't think these warnings preclude their use. The first is a concern for toxicity to cartilage. Theoretically, steroids and the local anesthetic that is usually injected with them can advance cartilage wear. Studies looking at this are inconclusive. Do not get cortisone injections more often than every three months in one knee to help mitigate this risk. Secondly, diabetics will likely see their blood sugars rise for the first two to three days after injection. This is also not a reason to proceed, just something to be aware of. Third, an uncommon side effect of steroids is what is known as a *steroid flare*. This is an intense swelling and pain within the knee that occurs for one to two days after steroid injection. Should this occur, contact the provider who gave the injection. The typical treatments are anti-inflammatory medications, ice, and time.

I believe the risks listed are low, and it's rare that we see adverse events following cortisone injections. I give cortisone injections liberally in my practice and abide strictly by the **Three-Month Rule.**

> **Cortisone Injections – The Three-Month Rule**
> - The effect typically lasts three months or less
> - Do not get one more frequently than every three months in the same knee
> - No injections within three months of surgery (on that knee)

> **Hyaluronic Acid Injections**
>
> **Recommendation:** YES—second-line treatment; and only for those with mild or moderate osteoarthritis. Not recommended for patients with severe arthritis.
>
> **Risk**: Low to moderate (see below for a description of risks). Note that these injections may not be covered by some insurance companies.

Hyaluronic acid is a gel-like substance that occurs naturally in the *synovial fluid* (knee fluid). Research has shown that this substance breaks down in the presence of osteoarthritis. These are also known as *viscosupplementation injections*, or patients refer to them as 'lubricating injections' or 'rooster comb injections' because some manufacturers have used rooster or chicken combs as a source of the substance. In theory, these injections might increase lubrication, increase shock absorption, and decrease inflammation to some degree. They can be given in a series of injections one week apart, or as a single injection, depending on the manufacturer.

The results of studies on hyaluronic acid injections are mixed. Medicare and some other insurance companies will still pay for these injections, which they typically will not do in the absence of quality scientific evidence demonstrating efficacy. On the other hand, the 2013 AAOS Guidelines state a strong recommendation AGAINST the use of hyaluronic acid injections for patients with symptomatic osteoarthritis of the knee.[2] The American College of Rheumatology has some confusing recommendations on these injections, but my interpretation is that they only recommend it in select patients and NOT as first-line treatment.[3] Some studies have been published since 2013 that show more promising results, especially in patients with milder arthritis.

There are some risks to note with hyaluronic acid injections. Standard risks of infection apply just as with steroid injections. I also caution patients that many will experience no improvement in symptoms, which is the primary reason it's a second-line treatment. For those who do see improvement, the relief might last six months to a year in some cases. This contrasts with steroid injections whereby more patients get relief, but it is often short-lived. Do not try these injections during an osteoarthritis *flare*, or in a knee with significant swelling. Steroids are better in those scenarios to knock down inflammation. Some patients will experience an increase in pain for the first several days after hyaluronic acid injections so be aware of that.

These injections should be used selectively, and ONLY in patients with osteoarthritis on the milder end of the spectrum. I don't give them more often than every six months in the same knee, and never within three months of a proposed surgery date.

---

### Platelet Rich Plasma (PRP) Injections

**Recommendation:** YES—second-line treatment; and only for those with mild or moderate osteoarthritis. Not recommended for patients with severe osteoarthritis.

**Risk**: Low to moderate (see below for a description of risks). Note that these injections are typically not covered by insurance.

---

Blood is composed of both cells and fluid (plasma). Both the cells and the plasma contain substances with healing potential. Technology has been developed to extract platelets and plasma from blood. This concentrated product is then injected into the knee with some theoretical ability to heal tissues and provide symptom relief.

Studies show mixed results on efficacy, with no high-level scientific evidence to support the use of PRP in the knee. The American Association of Hip and Knee Surgeons (AAHKS) specifically recommends against PRP use for advanced arthritis.[4] PRP has been marketed as a tool for sports injury treatment, which has increased its popularity in the absence of high-quality evidence. Those studies that support the use of PRP show small improvements in knee pain for up to a year after injection and primarily in patients with milder disease. No studies have shown that PRP injections slow progression of arthritis or re-grow cartilage.

PRP injections have some risk and controversy surrounding their use. One issue is that there are a lot of formulations that fall under the broad term of PRP. Some formulations are better than others. Aside from unknown efficacy, one of the biggest risks is cost. Most insurance companies do not cover them, so the cost to the patient can be up to $1000 per injection.

PRP is a reasonable second-line treatment option, but patients should be aware of the lack of high-level evidence, the cost of injections, and the potential that they do not get relief. Research shows that *leukocyte-reduced* formulations should be used in the knee.

### Stem Cell Injections

**Recommendation:** NO—currently there are too many problems with formulations, advertising, and research behind stem cell therapies to recommend their routine use for knee osteoarthritis.

**Risk**: High (see below for a description of risks)

Cell therapies are described as the process of taking living cells from a source and injecting them into another site with the idea that they will act on the delivery site to promote repair or regeneration. Beyond that definition, it is difficult to describe what constitutes *stem cell* therapies simply because the term is being used by patients, medical providers, and researchers to describe a wide range of treatments. *Stem cells* can be thought of as raw materials that can change into different types of more specialized cells in the body. The idea that a cell can be injected into a damaged environment and change into a specialized reparative or restorative cell is extremely attractive. This is an area of medicine that has a massive potential to cure disease.

The potential of stem cells and the current efficacy of injecting them into the knee joint with intended results are two different stories. There are significant problems that surround the topic of stem cell research and administration. The first is that there are a wide variety of different formulations being called "stem cells". The source of these cells could be humans, animals, amniotic fluid, umbilical cord cells, bone marrow, fat, muscle, or other sources. There is further confusion and variation in how these cells are processed before injection. Because of the wide variation in different formulations, there is a call in the scientific community to standardize language around these formulations for purposes of both research and clinical use.

The studies that surround stem cell injections for knee arthritis in humans are mixed, of low quality, and low in numbers. In my opinion, we are nowhere close to data that makes this a legitimate main-stream treatment. The AAHKS and AAOS have a position statement specifically recommending against stem cell injections for advanced hip and knee arthritis. According to AAHKS, "there is no data to support the idea that stem cells can sense the environment into which they are injected and repair damaged tissue."[4]

Stem cell and regenerative medicine clinics are a primary example of how marketing and hype can override science in the public's perception of quality treatment options. Stem cells have become a $45 billion industry, and the public is paying large cash payments, sometimes more than $5000 per injection, for this unproven treatment. There is no insurance company in the United States that currently covers these injections because of the cost and lack of evidence. The FDA has submitted warnings about certain formulations, and the Federal Trade Commission has fined stem cell clinics for false advertising. As of the writing of this book, unless they are injected by an academic center that is studying and publishing outcomes for stem cell treatments, I believe that injection of stem cells for knee arthritis is inappropriate.

I list this as a high-risk treatment because of all the

unknowns that surround the injections, the lack of high-quality research, the false advertising behind them, and the high cost to patients. Although I hope that someday we will have better research and formulations that deliver the potential and promise of stem cells, I currently recommend strongly against them.

> ### Prolotherapy
>
> **Recommendation:** NO—currently there are not enough high-quality research studies to recommend use.
>
> **Risk**: Low to moderate

Prolotherapy is a relatively new treatment that injects a sugar solution (like dextrose) into a patient's knee with the idea that the solution will irritate the joint surfaces and promote a healing response.

There have been several studies that show pain relief or improvement in function from this therapy. Most are of low quality. Larger, higher-quality studies are needed. I admit that recent studies show that this treatment has potential. I'm awaiting more studies and the support of any of the major orthopedic or rheumatologic medical associations before recommending this treatment.

## Chapter 5 Review

- Injections are an important treatment option for knee arthritis.
- It is important that patients understand the efficacy and risks of each treatment.
- All injections carry with them a low risk of introducing bacteria into the joint space.
- Avoid any injections into the knee joint if you are planning surgery within three months.
- Cortisone = steroid = corticosteroid injections can be beneficial for short-term pain relief and have a low to moderate risk profile.
- PRP injections should be considered only in patients with milder arthritis, should be considered second-line treatments, and often require the patient to pay outside of insurance.
- Stem cell injections currently have many problems in their formulations, research, advertising, and cost. There is not enough scientific evidence to justify the risk and cost of these injections.
- Prolotherapy has some promising studies but currently not enough high-level data to recommend it as a treatment option.

Chapter Six

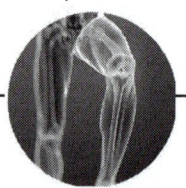

# Medications and Supplements

*Medications* are regulated by the FDA and are intended to treat or prevent medical conditions. They are widely available; many without a prescription.

*Supplements* are not regulated by the FDA and are considered non-pharmaceutical supplements to diet. They come in the form of concentrates, extracts, capsules, tablets, liquids, and powders. There is far less regulation and less scientific study surrounding supplements compared to medications.

This chapter will cover the most commonly used medications and supplements that are taken *orally* (by mouth) for the treatment of knee osteoarthritis.

> **Non-steroidal Anti-Inflammatory Drugs (NSAIDs)**
>
> **Recommendation:** YES—first-line treatment, but only in certain patients
>
> **Risk**: Moderate, especially if taken long-term (see cautions below)

NSAIDs are a class of medications that include both over-the-counter (OTC) and prescription varieties. These medications work on inflammation pathways in the body and function as pain relievers and fever reducers.

The common over-the-counter NSAIDs include ibuprofen (Advil® or Motrin®), naproxen (Aleve®), and aspirin. Ibuprofen and naproxen are the most commonly used NSAIDs for knee arthritis. Aspirin is less commonly used because of its potential for side effects when taken in higher doses.

Prescription NSAIDs come in many forms. They are generally more potent and have more side effects than the OTC variety.

| NSAID Side Effects and Cautions – IMPORTANT! |
|---|
| <ul><li>Risk of stomach ulcers</li><li>Risk of kidney impairment</li><li>Cardiovascular risks: heart, stroke, death</li><li>Increased risk of bleeding</li><li>Consult your physician before use if you have a history of any of the above conditions, high blood pressure, cardiovascular disease, are taking blood thinners, or plan to take NSAIDs for more than one week</li><li>All risks go up with higher doses and longer duration of use</li></ul> |

Between OTC and prescription versions, I suggest patients start with naproxen (first choice) or ibuprofen (second choice). These are generally safe, effective, and cheap medications. Check with your primary care doctor or pharmacist on dosing for you. Naproxen has a slight advantage over ibuprofen because it can be taken every twelve hours (versus every six to eight hours), and some studies show a slightly better effect in patients with knee arthritis pain. Some patients prefer ibuprofen over naproxen, so I would endorse ibuprofen in those patients.

NSAIDs are excellent pain relievers and are considered safe for healthy patients who take them for short periods of time (<30 days), intermittently, and in the lowest effective dose. However, there are some significant side effects and cautions to be aware of. Regular use increases the risk of stomach ulcers or stomach pains and they can impair kidney function. We usually recommend a medication to protect the stomach if patients are using NSAIDs regularly. Studies have shown an increased risk of death, heart attack, heart failure, and stroke if taken regularly. Some increase the risk of bleeding and should not be taken with blood-thinning medications or a history of bleeding. You should discontinue use with any stomach pains, bleeding, bruising, or other concerns related to these risks. All risks increase with prolonged use and higher doses. Consider alternating doses with NSAIDs and acetaminophen (Tylenol®). A safe bet is to let your primary care doctor know if you are going to be taking NSAIDs regularly.

More information on NSAIDs can be found on the FDA website: https://www.fda.gov/drugs/postmarket-drug-safety-information-patients-and-providers/nonsteroidal-anti-inflammatory-drugs-nsaids

> ### Acetaminophen (Tylenol®)
>
> **Recommendation:** YES–first-line treatment, but not in patients with liver disease
>
> **Risk**: Low

Acetaminophen became popular in the mid-1900s and has become a staple of pain management throughout the world. It has stood the test of time as a relatively safe and effective pain medication and fever reducer.

Acetaminophen is not an anti-inflammatory medication like the NSAIDs. It controls pain through different pathways. Studies have shown that it is not as effective as NSAIDs in controlling pain. The AAOS has labeled its recommendation for acetaminophen for knee arthritis as "inconclusive".[2] Its popularity remains because of its favorable safety profile and because it works *synergistically* with some other pain medications, meaning it enhances the effects of other medications.

Acetaminophen is a great first-line treatment for patients. It works for some better than others. It is also a great alternative for patients who cannot take NSAIDs. The biggest caution with acetaminophen is that it is cleared by the liver. Liver toxicity can occur if recommended doses are exceeded. A dose of 4,000 mg per 24-hour period should not be exceeded by any patient, and some patients should not exceed 3,000 mg in 24 hours. Discuss dosing for you with your primary care doctor or pharmacist. It should never be taken with alcohol and should be avoided by patients with liver disease.

## Opioid Pain Medications

**Recommendation:** NO—you should avoid opioid pain medications for osteoarthritis pain.

**Risk**: High

These are prescription-only medications. Commonly prescribed opioids include oxycodone (Percocet® or Oxycontin®), hydrocodone (Norco® or Vicodin®), morphine (MS Contin®), hydromorphone (Dilaudid®), and tramadol (Ultram®).

Opioids are excellent short-term pain relievers that come at a significant cost in terms of side effects and addictive potential. It's no secret that the United States is in the midst of an opioid crisis. We consume the majority of the world's opioid supply despite accounting for 5 percent of the world's population. Opioid addiction, abuse, and deaths occur at staggering rates. I see more side effects and problems associated with opioid pain medications than any other type of medication used in my practice. Common side effects include mood swings, itching, sweating, constipation, nausea, vomiting, dry mouth, confusion, dizziness, hallucinations, urinary retention, and insomnia. If taken in high doses, they can cause respiratory depression and death.

Although they are excellent short-term pain relievers, opioids are terrible long-term pain relievers. The body develops not only a chemical dependence on them, but also a tolerance for them. Over time, the body's receptors become more sensitive to pain. This means after exposure to opioids, everything might hurt MORE (not less), a response called *opioid-induced hyperalgesia*. The body then requires even more opioids to achieve pain control and the cycle repeats. This is the crux and the tragedy of opioid addiction.

AAHKS has a clear position statement on opioids: "It is our position that the use of opioids for the treatment of osteoarthritis of the hip and knee should be avoided and reserved for only for exceptional circumstances."[5] Don't use them for arthritis pain. If you are on them, talk with your primary care doctor about how to get off them. They have more negative effects on your health and wellbeing than you may be aware of. If you have surgery and need them for pain control, use them for the shortest duration possible.

> ### Duloxetine
>
> **Recommendation:** YES—third-line treatment, and only for patients unable or unwilling to undergo other treatments.
>
> **Risk**: Low

Duloxetine is a prescription medication that's part of a family of drugs used primarily to treat depression and anxiety, but also has some uses for treating chronic pain. I include it for two reasons. First, there is a conditional recommendation for its use by the American College of Rheumatology.[3] This is not a medication I prescribe, but there are some good randomized studies showing that duloxetine decreases chronic pain from knee arthritis. Secondly, it is an alternative for chronic pain relief in those patients who have severe arthritis pain but are not able or willing to undergo other treatments like knee replacement. Duloxetine is not for everyone and has side effects, so discuss it with your primary care doctor if you are interested.

> ### Supplements
>
> **Recommendation:** NO—none are effective for knee osteoarthritis. Take supplements only if your doctor prescribes them for other health reasons.
>
> **Risk**: Unknown since formulations are not monitored or controlled

As we move on to supplements, I want to emphasize again that supplements are a tricky subject when it comes to treating medical conditions. Supplements are intended to add to our normal diet and not treat diseases, however, our society has "medicinized" supplements – meaning we are encouraged to use them like medications. Many patients believe whole-heartedly that supplements are better for them than medicines.

The primary problem with supplements is that the FDA is not monitoring them. When you purchase a supplement, there is little to no regulation with regard to quality or quantity. We have romanticized the supplement world and probably overuse them as a society.

As a rule, there are <u>no supplements</u> that are proven to be effective in treating knee osteoarthritis or preventing the advancement of osteoarthritis. None. This comes as a surprise to many patients who have been taking supplements for years to either "save" their joints or to alleviate joint pain. Eating a healthy diet, keeping your body mass index in the recommended range, and exercising regularly will do far more for you than any supplement.

The best known and most commonly consumed supplements for arthritis are glucosamine and chondroitin, and I will address them separately below. Any of the other so-called osteoarthritis supplements lack scientific evidence to support use for osteoarthritis pain including:

- Turmeric/curcumin
- Avocado soybean unsaponfiables (ASU)
- MSM (Methylsulfonylmethane)
- Collagen
- Rose hip
- Willow bark extract
- Omega-3 fatty acids

### Glucosamine / Chondroitin

**Recommendation:** NO

**Risk:** Unknown since formulations are not monitored or controlled

In the 1990s, I recall a family member who recommended glucosamine and chondroitin to me for knee pain. In the early 2000s, there were some studies showing that certain formulations might be beneficial. The scientific evidence now seems clear that glucosamine and chondroitin should no longer be recommended for osteoarthritis pain. The American Academy of Orthopaedic Surgeons cites "strong evidence" against the use of glucosamine and chondroitin.[2] The American College of Rheumatology also recommends against both. [3] A surprising number of patients still come to my clinic believing that they are protecting their joints by taking these supplements.

The studies seem clear that both glucosamine and chondroitin are safe substances to ingest. The problem is that when you purchase a supplement containing one or both, there is no way to know if you are taking what you think you are taking. I recommend that you save your money and focus on other treatments.

### Calcium and Vitamin D

**Recommendation:** YES–but NOT for arthritis pain

**Risk**: Low

I'm including some recommendations for calcium and vitamin D NOT because they treat arthritis pain, but because they are important for your bone and joint health. A common point of confusion exists between *osteoarthritis* and *osteoporosis*. Osteoporosis refers to decreased bone density that occurs as a natural part of aging, which is more pronounced in females than males. Patients with decreased bone density have an increased risk of fracture. This is different from joint surface wear we see in osteoarthritis.

Calcium and vitamin D have several benefits within the body including slowing bone loss, reducing blood pressure and cholesterol levels, and they may help prevent tooth loss. Current recommendations for both are below. Discuss these dosages with your doctor. Dosages provided include **DIET + SUPPLEMENTS**:

- Premenopausal women and men: 1000 mg calcium and 600 IU vitamin D daily
- Postmenopausal women: 1200 mg calcium and 800 IU vitamin D daily
- You should not exceed 2000 mg of calcium per day due to the risk of side effects

- Foods high in calcium: dairy products, soymilk, and dark/leafy vegetables
- Sources of vitamin D: fish, mushrooms, and sunlight (skin exposure)

## Chapter 6 Review

- Medications are controlled and monitored by the FDA; supplements are not.
- Never exceed the recommended dosages of medications and let your primary care doctor know about any medications you are going to take for more than a week at a time.
- NSAIDs tend to work well for osteoarthritis pain, but you need to be aware of the risks and side effects.
- Acetaminophen is generally not quite as effective as NSAIDs for arthritis pain, but it has a more favorable safety profile.
- Opioids are recommended for arthritis pain ONLY in rare circumstances.
- Duloxetine has some potential to relieve arthritis pain.
- There are no supplements known to prevent or treat knee osteoarthritis effectively.
- Calcium and vitamin D are important supplements for bone density but are not used to treat arthritis

Chapter Seven

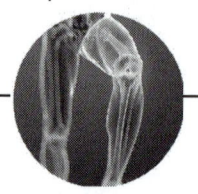

# Topical Creams, Rubs, and Ointments

Topical therapies are medications that are applied to the skin over the knee joint with the intended effect of pain reduction. All of the therapies listed can be purchased over-the-counter with the exception of some topical NSAIDs.

> **Topical Therapies**
>
> **Recommendation:** YES—first-line treatment.
>
> **Risk**: Low

Topical therapies are recommended not because I believe the effect is dramatic. Any pain relief from these treatments is expected to be mild. I recommend them because they are generally safe and low-cost options. If patients experience pain relief from these treatments, the duration of effect is short. They are not definitive treatment options for advanced knee arthritis and should be used in combination with other treatments.

Topical capsaicin is safe, effective, and has been shown in some studies to be more effective than placebo for treatment of knee osteoarthritis. It causes a burning sensation due to the active ingredient in hot peppers. A glove is recommended for application to avoid burning of the hand. Capsaicin affects the way pain messages are transmitted in local tissues, and it can take a week or two of daily application to accomplish this.

Topical over-the-counter salicylates are similar to aspirin. These over-the-counter creams and ointments are best known by their trade names Bengay® and Aspercreme®. Usually, a substance such as menthol is added to it which provides the cooling sensation and familiar smell. There is little research demonstrating effectiveness for arthritis pain. Since some of the salicylates are absorbed into the body, you should consult a doctor before regular use if you are on blood thinners.

Sometimes camphor or menthol are used as the primary ingredient in creams and rubs. Common products that use these are Icy Hot® and Biofreeze®. There is little research into these, but also little risk in trying them.

Topical NSAIDs are available by prescription. Some research has shown them to be effective for arthritis pain. These have the potential to have some of the same side effects as their oral counterparts, however, the amount of mediation absorbed is less than oral NSAIDs. Since they require a prescription, your medical provider can help decide if they are right for you.

## Chapter 7 Review

- Topical treatments are generally safe and effective alternatives for knee arthritis.
- They are unlikely to provide long-term relief for advanced knee arthritis.
- Multiple formulations are available over-the-counter
- Consult your medical provider if you would like to try topical NSAIDs

Chaper Eight

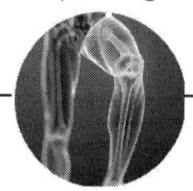

# Braces and Assistive Devices

Braces and assistive devices are intended to affect the way the way the knee is loaded. The idea is that if we can change the way weight is distributed through the knee joint, we can change pain symptoms.

> ### Knee Braces
>
> **Recommendation:** YES–third-line treatment. Braces are worth trying for those who have limited options but be aware they don't work for everyone.
>
> **Risk**: Low

I believe braces have a role in treating knee arthritis for patients who either don't want surgery or cannot tolerate other options. There are two types that may help arthritis pain. The first is the neoprene knee sleeve which can be purchased in drug stores and sporting goods stores. Neoprene is the material that wetsuits are made from. Look for a style with no hinges or metal in it. Some might have some Velcro straps as shown in Figure 8-1. I prefer the kind with a hole cut out around the patella in the front. While scientific evidence is lacking showing significant pain relief, I think they help keep the knee warm (less pain), keep knee swelling down (less pain), and make the knee feel more stable.

The second type of knee brace I've used is the *unloader brace*. These are typically prescription braces that are more expensive than a knee sleeve. The idea behind unloader braces is that they push a *varus* or *valgus* knee (see Chapter 2 if you need to review these terms), so that the most worn part of the knee is unloaded. Studies behind unloader braces are inconclusive. I prescribe them when patients want to avoid surgery and are looking for a treatment option. My own experience is that they help less than half of the patients who try them, so this is not a strong recommendation.

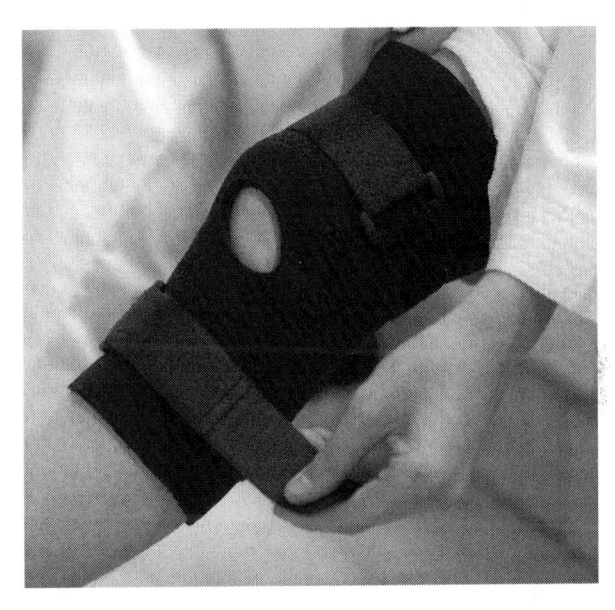

**Figure 8-1**: Simple neoprene knee sleeve

### Shoe Inserts

**Recommendation:** NO–due to lack of convincing scientific data

**Risk**: Low

Shoe inserts are covered because patients ask about them and they have been historically used by many orthopedic surgeons. I admit I had little exposure to them in training or practice, and I've never had a patient tell me that any type of shoe insert helped with their knee pain.

Shoe inserts come in two varieties: insoles and heel wedges. Insoles are the type of insert that fills most of the shoe and might even replace a shoe's stock insole. I would also lump orthotics into this category. I'm not aware of any high-quality studies showing that insoles or orthotics significantly affect knee arthritis pain.

The second type is heel wedges. Wedges are made to change the angle of the foot, and therefore the angle of the knee and where the knee is loaded. The American Academy of Orthopaedic Surgeons lists a moderate recommendation against the use of heel wedges.[2] I additionally have some concerns about changing the angle of the foot and ankle to decrease knee pain.

> **Cane, Crutches, Walker, or Wheelchair**
>
> **Recommendation:** YES—first-line treatment if unable to walk safely or comfortably otherwise
>
> **Risk:** Low

Patients regularly show up in my knee arthritis clinic using these devices. There are two reasons to consider one of these assistive devices. A primary reason to avoid falls. A fall from either loss of balance or a buckling knee can cause problems more significant than knee arthritis. The second reason to use one is to offload the knee joint due to pain.

Which you choose depends on the severity of symptoms. Most patients choose a cane or walker over crutches. Walkers come in many varieties. Some have wheels, brakes, and even a seat to stop and rest. Visit your local medical supply store or search the Internet for options. A wheelchair should be reserved for patients who cannot walk safely or comfortably across a room.

> **Kinesiology Taping**
>
> **Recommendation:** NO
>
> **Risk:** Low

Kinesiology taping has become trendy in the world of sports and therapy. Athlete testimonials have probably driven this more than science. As stated in Chapter 4, I believe in therapists and the work they do for our patients. Our opinions diverge on this subject, as many therapists suggest taping much more frequently than physicians. This is a treatment with no-high quality studies to support it. The American Academy of Orthopaedic Surgeons has no position or information available on patellar taping, and the American College of Rheumatology conditionally recommends it only for patients who have moderate or severe arthritis and are unwilling or unable to undergo knee replacement surgery.[3]

The theory behind taping for arthritis pain is flawed. There is significant mobility between the skin and underlying muscles, tendons, and other structures that are supposed to be affected by the taping. The idea that an externally applied tape can change mechanics of underlying structures, lift the skin, or decrease lymphatic fluid or inflammation is a bit hopeful. The major companies that sell these products have disclaimers on their websites stating that these treatments are not proven. My preference is to leave this out of treatment regimens and focus on treatments with better evidence.

## Chapter 8 Review

- All types of braces and assistive devices lack strong scientific evidence behind their treatment.

- Neoprene sleeves and unloader braces help some patients and are worth a try if other options are not available or effective.

- I recommend against shoe wedges and knee taping.

- A cane, crutch, walker, or wheelchair is an excellent idea if there is a risk of falling or pain is too great to walk without it.

Chapter Nine

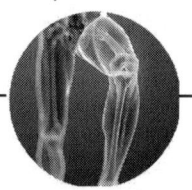

# Where to Go from Here

We have discussed the most common treatments available for knee arthritis. This is the point in time where you decide which combination of treatments best suits your needs. I encourage you to try different options. As everything about you is unique, so is the way your body will react to various knee treatments. This chapter has a few parting thoughts as you move forward.

## Be Skeptical

I don't mean that you should suspect that all medical providers are trying to deceive you. The doctor-patient relationship is founded on trust, so if you have a medical provider you know and trust, heed this advice. On the other hand, it's okay to ask for scientific evidence behind the treatments that are recommended to you, especially if they are not mainstream and ESPECIALLY if your insurance doesn't cover that treatment and you are paying out-of-pocket for them. It is our job as medical providers to offer patients *informed consent* before administering treatments. This means that you should know what the risks and benefits are, as well as the chance of it working based on large, well-designed studies. If those types of studies don't exist, you should know that before accepting the treatment.

## Use Credible Sources

Remember that there is no requirement for credibility to place a television, radio, magazine, and newspaper advertisement. These ads often use doctor or patient testimony to draw you in and make you think a treatment is credible. I urge you to ignore these when considering the best treatments for any health condition.

There are a few organizations that I trust when it comes to websites for knee arthritis that are listed in the Appendix. I believe that these organizations have the patients' best interests in mind when they develop patient education resources and guidelines.

After reading this book, I suggest discussing treatment options with your own primary care providers and/or orthopedic providers. If you don't have a primary care doctor, establish one. Your own providers can give guidance catered to your own personal needs and health conditions.

## When to Consider Surgery

Many patients I see have had the old "clean out" scope for their arthritic knee. There is no long-term benefit to cleaning out an arthritic knee with arthroscopy. Remember, arthritis is a condition, not a substance, so you can't really clean out worn cartilage and expect a good result because what's left is exposed bone and more worn cartilage. The exception here is that if patients have a meniscus tear that is causing *mechanical symptoms* (clicking, locking, catching) and pain, it may provide some relief. Discuss this with your local surgeon.

Knee replacement is generally reserved for patients who meet these five criteria:

- moderate to severe arthritis
- failed non-operative treatment options
- daily, life-limiting pain
- healthy enough for surgery
- understand the surgery, the risks, and the benefits

In our companion book *Your Knee Replacement* (OrthoSkool Publishing) as well as our website www.orthoskool.com, you will find a more in-depth discussion about knee replacement surgery, who typically qualifies, and what to expect with this procedure. Your local orthopedic surgeon is the best resource if you are wondering if this procedure is right for you.

## Chapter 9 Review

- It is okay to be skeptical of medical treatments that are not backed by science, are advertised and new and groundbreaking, and especially if you are asked to pay out-of-pocket for them.

- Use credible sources to research your conditions and then discuss them with your own medical team.

- Knee surgery should be reserved for patients who fail conservative measures. Your local orthopedic surgeon can discuss whether surgery is right for you.

# Appendix

## Strength Exercises for Knee Arthritis

The quadriceps and hamstring muscle groups are the primary dynamic stabilizers of the knee joint. Some muscles around the hip also play a role in stabilizing the knee and assist with gait. The following exercises focus on strengthening these muscle groups. Avoid exercises that increase pain in the knee.

**Quadriceps Isolation:** Using slow movements, move the knee through the arc of the motion shown. It is important to focus on squeezing your quadriceps muscle at the top of the arc (when the knee is fully straight). Hold the knee straight for three to five seconds, then go back down slowly. If the long arc version is painful or difficult, try one of the short arc variants. An ankle weight may be used to increase resistance. If these exercises are performed correctly, your thigh muscles should feel tired after fifteen repetitions. Aim for three sets of fifteen repetitions at least three days per week on each leg.

1. Long arc quadriceps strengthening: Sitting in a chair, table, or edge of an elevated bed, put the back of your knees against the edge of the sitting surface and move the knee slowly from bent to straight. Squeeze at the top!

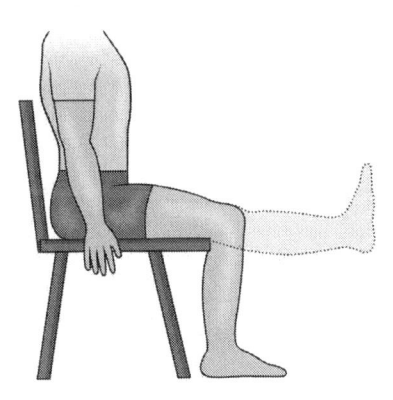

2. <u>Short arc quadriceps strengthening</u>: This is similar to the long arc version; however, the knee does not bend as far. Decreasing the bend puts less stress on your patellofemoral joint. You can do these in a chair or on the floor with a roll of towels under the knee as shown.

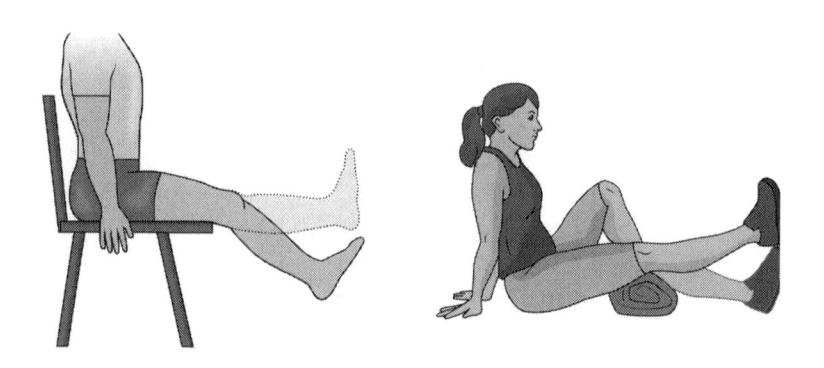

**Squats:** These strengthen both the quadriceps and the hamstrings. Do whichever variant is most comfortable for you.

1. <u>Standing squat</u>: With both arms extended outward for balance, try to keep your back upright and bend at the knees. Go down only as far as you can comfortably, but do not go past a 90-degree bend in the knees.

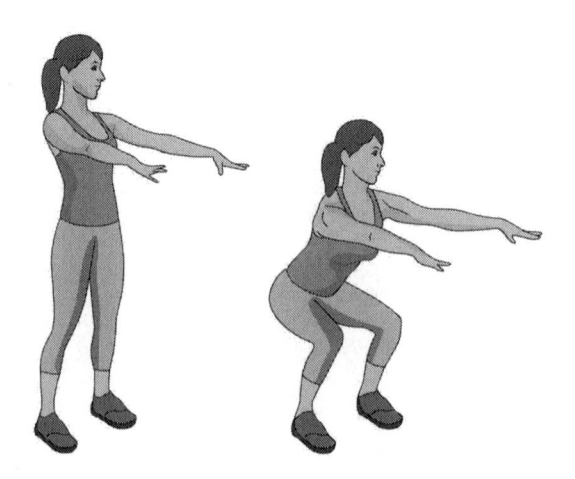

Appendix

<u>Chair assisted squat</u>: Some people find using a chair as a reference point helpful. Try not to fully sit down on the chair. Lower and tap buttocks on it, then return to standing. Higher chairs or a bed can decrease how far you need to bend your knees.

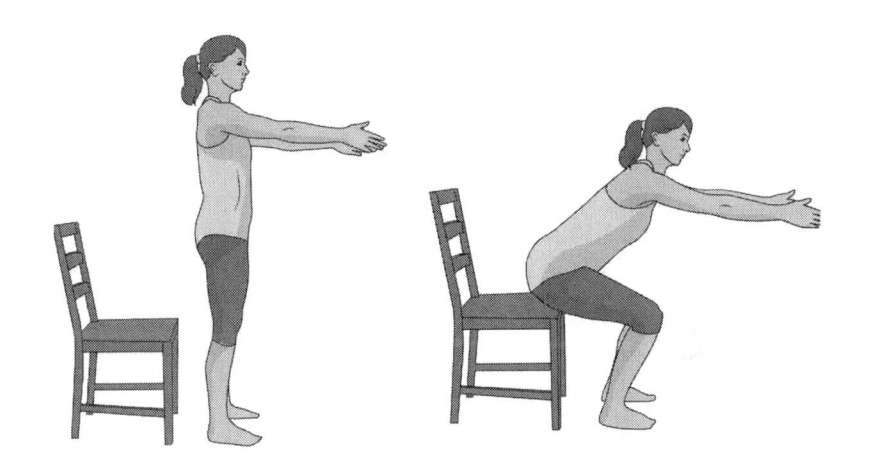

<u>Wall sits</u>: Using a wall for stabilization is easier for some patients than squatting up and down. Set goal times and increase as you get stronger.

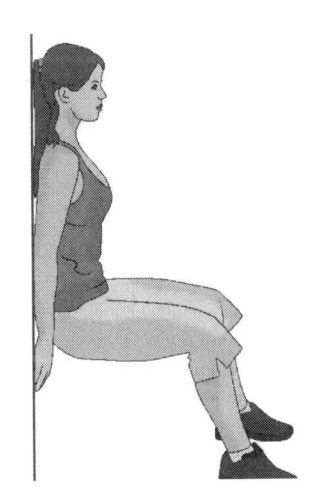

**Standing Hamstring Curls:** Using a chair or rail for balance, lift one foot off the ground so the knee is bent 90 degrees, hold a few seconds at the top, and return the foot to the floor. You can add ankle weights to increase resistance. Do three sets of fifteen curls for each leg at least three days per week.

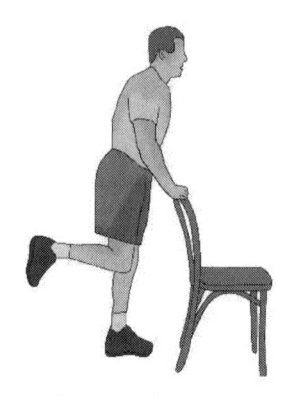

**Lateral Leg Lifts:** Lateral leg lifts can promote strength in some key muscles around the hip joint. Lying on your side, hold your leg straight and lift to an angle of 45 degrees with the ground, hold for two seconds, then lower your straight leg to the floor slowly. Aim for three sets of fifteen for each leg at least three days per week.

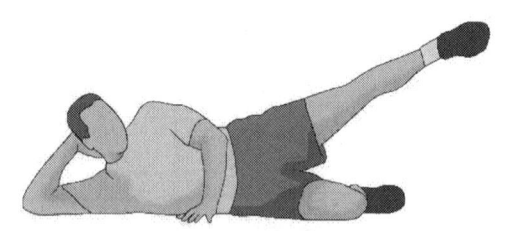

**Stationary Bike**: This is one of the best tools for strengthening the knee. It doesn't matter if you use the upright version (shown) or a recumbent bike. Riding bikes outdoors is also great, but the stationary bike provides a more controlled environment without traffic, hills, or risk of tipping over. I suggest the following progression of seat positions.

1. <u>High seat</u>: Start by putting the seat at the highest level where you can still (barely) reach the pedals on both sides without your pelvis rocking back and forth on the seat. This position helps get your knee fully extended and requires the least bend to make a full revolution. Ride three to five minutes in this position making slow revolutions with minimal resistance.

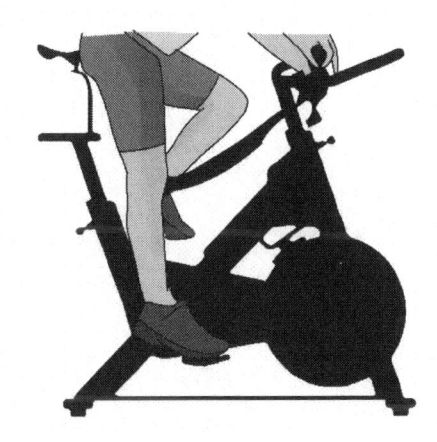

2. <u>Low seat</u>: Next, put the seat at the lowest level where you can still make a revolution with both knees. This position helps with knee flexion. Ride three to five minutes in this position with slow revolutions and minimal resistance.

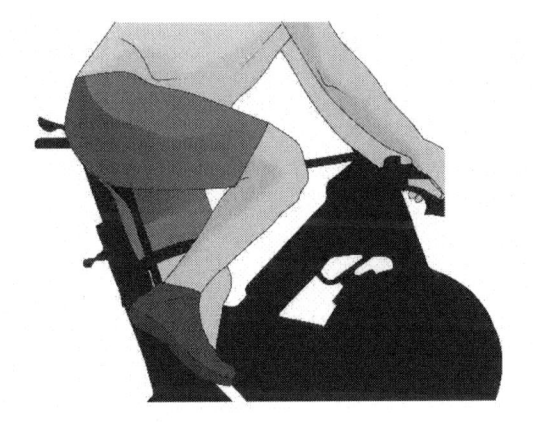

3. <u>Middle/comfortable seat</u>: The ideal seat height for normal riding yields about a 30-degree bend in the knee when you are at the very bottom of the pedal stroke. With the seat in this position, you should be able to make a full revolution without reaching too far at the bottom or bending the knee too much at the top of the pedal stroke. You can turn up the resistance so that your thigh muscles feel fatigued. Try to pedal at 90 revolutions per minute. Work up to thirty to sixty-minute sessions with resistance, three days per week.

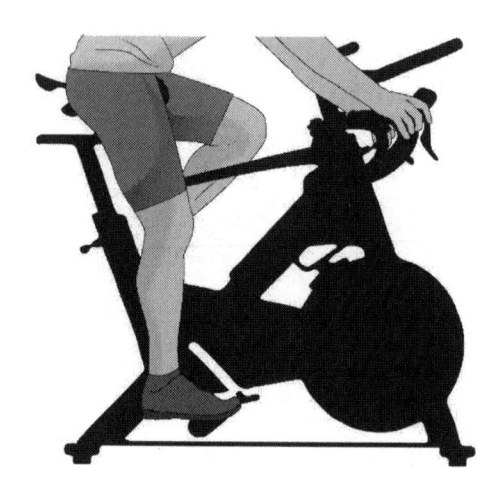

# Stretching Exercises for Knee Arthritis

It is helpful for most patients to stretch muscles that cross the knee joint. Stretching can improve flexibility and decrease knee pain. Remember that GENTLE stretching is the goal. Always consult a physical therapist if you have questions. All stretches can be held for 10-15 seconds, rest, and repeat for a total of two sets for each leg.

**Quadriceps Stretch:** Lying on your side, grab your foot and gently pull it toward your buttock. You should feel this in your thigh.

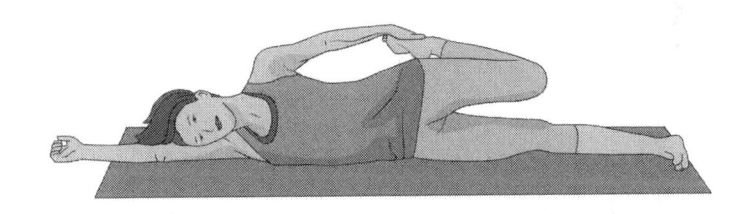

**Hamstrings Stretch:** Placing your foot on a stool, chair, or stair, keep your leg straight and bow toward your foot, decreasing the space between your chest and your thigh. You should feel this down the back of your extended leg. Bring your toes toward your head for an extra stretch.

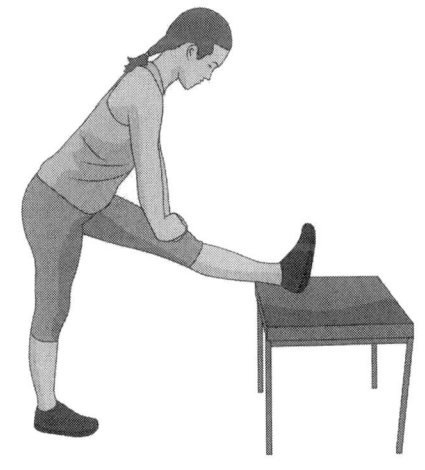

**Heel Cord Stretch:** This stretch works on your calf muscles and the strong tendons in your heel. You should feel it in the back of your leg from the knee to the foot. Try doing these with both a straight knee and a slightly bent knee to stretch different calf muscles.

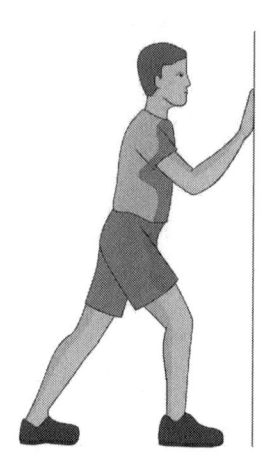

**IT Band Stretch:** Cross one leg over the other and reach over your head with the arm on the side of the back leg. Try to make a "C" with your body. You should feel this on the outside of your hip, thigh, and knee. Avoid this stretch if you have difficulty with balance.

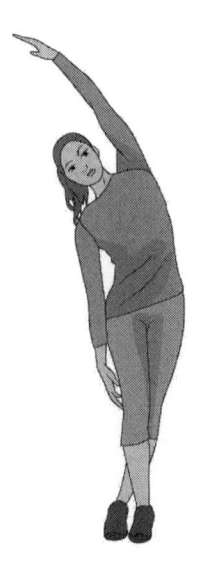

# Other Resources

## Knee Arthritis
### American Academy of Orthopaedic Surgeons (AAOS)
- The largest orthopedic organization in the world has an excellent patient education website that has hundreds of articles, videos, and other resources for bone and joint health: https://www.orthoinfo.org/

### American Association of Hip and Knee Surgeons (AAHKS)
- You can find a lot of valuable patient information on arthritis as well as hip and knee replacements: hipknee.aahks.org
- AAHKS as some position statements on topics like stem cell therapies and opioid use here: www.aahks.org/position-statements

### American College of Rheumatology (ACR)
- A high-quality resource on various types of arthritis, particularly inflammatory conditions such as rheumatoid arthritis: www.rheumatology.org/I-Am-A/Patient-Caregiver

## Mental Health and Meditation Books

*10% Happier* by Dan Harris, 2014.
If you are unfamiliar with meditation and mindfulness, this is an easy read and a great place to start.

*The Power of Now* by Eckhart Tolle, 1999.

Tolle is a visionary, teacher, and influential leader in the world of mindfulness. This book starts strong and then repeats some themes, but it has the potential to be life-changing.

*Cognitive Behavioral Therapy Made Simple* by Seth J. Gillihan, Ph.D., 2018.

There is some evidence that this type of therapy can help with post-operative pain. This book requires more effort than those listed above. It has strategies and exercises that may strengthen mental wellness and prepare you for surgery.

# Knee Arthritis Glossary

| | |
|---|---|
| **AAHKS** | American Association of Hip and Knee Surgeons |
| **AAOS** | American Academy of Orthopaedic Surgeons |
| **adipose tissue** | Fat tissue. |
| **anecdotal evidence** | A very low level of scientific evidence that supports the use of a particular treatment based on experience but in the absence of true scientific study or peer-reviewed publications. |
| **arthritis** | An inflamed joint, usually with pain. |
| **arthron** | A Greek word meaning "joint". |
| **arthroplasty** | A term that describes reshaping a joint, or what we commonly call joint replacement. |
| **articular cartilage** | Surface cartilage in the knee joint. This covers the ends of the femur, tibia, and patella. It provides a very smooth and slick surface to facilitate joint motion with low friction. |
| **articulate** | To form a joint. To rub together. |
| **autoimmune** | A disease whereby the body produces an inflammatory reaction against normal cells. |
| **body mass index** | A formula used to assess obesity that takes into account a patient's height and weight. |
| **bone on bone arthritis** | An x-ray finding where all the cartilage space is gone on x-ray, and bones normally separated by cartilage are touching each other. |
| **bronchitis** | Inflamed bronchi (tubes in the lungs). |

| | |
|---|---|
| **cartilage** | A substance found in joints that serves to protect the ends of two bones forming a joint. |
| **cartilage space narrowing** | Loss of cartilage space in the knee joint, seen on x-ray or other imaging studies. |
| **chronic** | A persistent or long-term condition (versus "acute" which describes a short-term condition). |
| **colitis** | An inflamed colon. |
| **compartments** | A distinct area of cartilage within the knee. The knee has three cartilage compartments that have different wear characteristics. |
| **corticosteroid** | See steroid. This is a synonym for steroid and cortisone. |
| **cortisone** | See steroid. This is a synonym for steroid and corticosteroid. |
| **deformity** | An optional feature of arthritis, whereby a joint is angulated due to underlying bone and cartilage wear. |
| **dynamic** | With motion. Dynamic stabilizers of the knee joint function with muscles and movement. |
| **expert opinion** | An article published in a medical journal that often lacks significant scientific evidence but represents the opinion of an expert in the field of study. |
| **extension** | How much your knee can straighten. |
| **femur** | The thigh bone. The longest bone in the body. |
| **fibula** | A long, thin bone in the lower leg that does not play a significant role in knee function or knee replacement surgery. |

| | |
|---|---|
| **flare** | A short-term but intense increase in arthritis pain and inflammation. |
| **flexion** | How much your knee bends. |
| **hemoglobin** | The substance in red blood cells that carries oxygen. The amount of hemoglobin is measurable with a lab test. |
| **hinge joint** | A joint that bends in only one plane like a door hinge. Examples are the knee and elbow. |
| **inflammation** | The body's local response to injury or wear that is typically associated with swelling, pain, and warmth. |
| **inflammatory arthritis** | A form of arthritis where the body causes abnormal inflammation in a joint, typically due to an underlying autoimmune disorder such as rheumatoid arthritis. |
| **inherent** | Things you are born with or cannot change. |
| **-itis** | A suffix used in medicine that means "inflammation". |
| **knee replacement** | A surgical procedure where the surfaces within the knee joint are replaced with metal and plastic. |
| **lateral** | Away from the midline of the body. The lateral compartment of the knee is the one farthest away from the midline. |
| **ligaments** | Strong, fibrous, soft tissue structures that connect two bones together. |
| **mechanical symptoms** | Symptoms in the knee that include catching, locking, or clicking. |
| **medial** | Toward the midline of the body. The medial compartment of the knee is the one closest to the midline. |

| | |
|---|---|
| **medical clearance** | A less desirable term for the medical optimization process that occurs around the time of surgery. |
| **medications** | Chemical compounds that are regulated by the FDA and used for the purpose treating diseases or symptoms. |
| **menisci** | The plural form of meniscus. |
| **meniscus** | A c-shaped cartilage disk in the knee that helps to cushion the joint and protect the underlying articular cartilage surfaces. |
| **mild arthritis** | Mild inflammation or minimal cartilage space narrowing in a joint, usually, but not always, associated with mild symptoms. |
| **mindfulness** | A state of living whereby we guide ourselves to live in the moment. |
| **moderate arthritis** | A condition in between mild and severe arthritis. Typically, at least half of the cartilage space is gone on x-ray. |
| **modifiable** | Things you can change. |
| **multifactorial** | Many factors contribute to a condition. |
| **myths** | Medical treatments that lack verifiable scientific evidence to support their use but are still used by patients and some medical practitioners. |
| **NSAIDs** | Non-steroidal anti-inflammatory drugs (examples are ibuprofen and naproxen). |
| **occupational therapist** | A therapist that has expertise in performing activities of daily living and self-care after surgery. |
| **opioid-induced hyperalgesia** | A phenomenon that occurs when patients are exposed to opioid pain medications and pain receptors become more sensitive to pain over time. |

| | |
|---|---|
| **osteoarthritis** | The most common form of arthritis, typically described as "wear and tear" arthritis. |
| **osteophytes** | Bone spurs. |
| **osteoporosis** | Decreased density of the bones which occurs naturally with age, more prominent in females than males. |
| **pain** | An optional feature of arthritis. Not every joint with arthritis has pain. |
| **patella** | The kneecap. |
| **patellofemoral compartment** | The compartment of the knee that includes only the patella and the trochlea. |
| **patient testimonies** | Individual patients provide testimony that a particular treatment was effective for them. |
| **peer-reviewed** | A scientific study that has been reviewed by a professional peer with expertise in the subject matter of that study. This is done before publication in medical journals. |
| **placebo effect** | A commonly accepted effect that occurs only the idea of a treatment has the proposed effect of the treatment. |
| **prehab** | Physical therapy that occurs before a surgical procedure. |
| **primary care provider** | Also known as a PCP. This is a general practitioner that looks after your overall health condition. This might be a doctor, nurse practitioner, or physician assistant. |
| **randomized control trial** | A scientific study wherein the researchers take a treatment, randomly assign that treatment to a group of patients, and gave an alternative or treatment to other patients, and analyze the results. |

| | |
|---|---|
| **rheumatoid arthritis** | The most common type of inflammatory arthritis whereby the body attacks its own cells, creating an inflammatory response and wear of cartilage. |
| **severe arthritis** | Severe inflammation or severe cartilage space narrowing in a joint, usually, but not always, associated with severe symptoms. |
| **static** | Without motion. Static stabilizers of the knee joint don't require muscles to function. |
| **stem cells** | Cells with the potential to develop into many different types of cells in the body. |
| **steroid** | A class of medications used to decrease inflammation and pain. There are oral and injectable forms. Synonyms include corticosteroid and cortisone. |
| **supplements** | Non-pharmaceutical dietary aids that are not regulated by the FDA. |
| **symptomatic relief** | Addressing the symptoms of a disease without fixing the underlying problem or changing the underlying structure. |
| **synergistically** | Two drugs working in a cooperative manner to produce a result greater than either drug would produce individually. |
| **tendons** | Fibrous soft tissue structures that connect muscles to bones. |
| **tibia** | The shin bone. The top of the tibia is part of the knee joint. |
| **total knee replacement** | All three compartments of the knee are replaced with metal and plastic joint surfaces. |

| | |
|---|---|
| **trochlea** | A cartilage-covered groove in the femur where the patella slides up and down. |
| **uni** | A synonym for unicompartmental knee arthroplasty. |
| **unicompartmental knee arthroplasty** | A knee replacement procedure where only one compartment of the knee joints is replaced with metal and plastic joint surfaces. |
| **valgus** | Knock-kneed deformity in the knee joint. |
| **varus** | Bowlegged deformity in the knee joint. |
| **viscosupplementation injections** | Hyaluronic acid injections |

# Image Credits

Figure 1-1   © [martialred] / Adobe Stock
Figure 2-4   © [rob3000] / Adobe Stock
Figure 2-5   © [apfelweile] and [stockdevil] / Adobe Stock
Figure 2-6   © [kintarapong] / Adobe Stock
Figure 8-1   © [Andriy Petrenko] / Adobe Stock

Stationary bike images in Appendix © [barbulat] / Adobe Stock.

Uncredited images are either owned by the Publisher or were obtained from stock image sources that do not require crediting. All images in this book are subject to applicable copyright law.

## Selected References

1. *Executive Summary of Physical Activity Guidelines for Americans, 2nd edition.* 2019; Available from: https://health.gov/paguidelines/second-edition/pdf/PAG_ExecutiveSummary.pdf.

2. Brown, G.A., *AAOS clinical practice guideline: treatment of osteoarthritis of the knee: evidence-based guideline, 2nd edition.* J Am Acad Orthop Surg, 2013. 21(9): p. 577-9.

3. Hochberg, M.C., et al., *American College of Rheumatology 2012 recommendations for the use of nonpharmacologic and pharmacologic therapies in osteoarthritis of the hand, hip, and knee.* Arthritis Care Res (Hoboken), 2012. 64(4): p. 465-74.

4. *Biologics for Advanced Hip and Knee Arthritis - Position of the American Association of Hip and Knee Surgeons.* Available from: http://www.aahks.org/position-statements/biologics-for-advanced-hip-and-knee-arthritis/.

5. *Opioid Use for the Treatment of Osteoarthritis of the Hip and Knee - Position of the American Association of Hip and Knee Surgeons.* Available from: http://www.aahks.org/position-statements/opioid-use-for-the-treatment-of-osteoarthritis-of-the-hip-and-knee/.

# Are you interested in information on knee or hip replacement surgery?

Check out these websites for an engaging, interactive, online education experience:

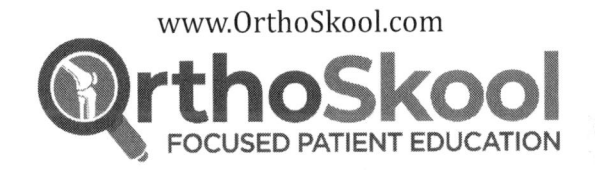

www.OrthoSkool.com

**OrthoSkool**
FOCUSED PATIENT EDUCATION

www.KneeSkool.com

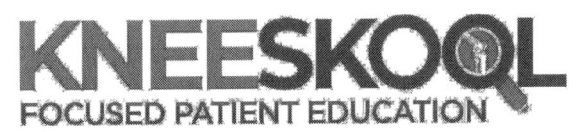

**KNEESKOOL**
FOCUSED PATIENT EDUCATION

www.HipSkool.com

**HIPSKOOL**
FOCUSED PATIENT EDUCATION

Manufactured by Amazon.ca
Bolton, ON